Unlocking
Hidden Health Secrets in the
Bible

Judy Savoy, Ph.D.

Unlocking Health Secrets in the Bible
By Judy Savoy, Ph.D.

ISBN-13:
978-1497462281

ISBN-10:
1497462282

Printed in the United States of America

Dedication

This book is dedicated to all true seekers of physical and mental health, as well as to those desiring a closer relationship with the Almighty One.

Acknowledgments

I wish to thank Tamara Luchini, Marcia Montgomery, Brenda Kaneshiro, and Paula Montgomery for their editorial suggestions; Ruth Phillingane and Dr. Livia Forbes for their medical input; my daughter Jill Rodriguez, for her encouragement and support; and my son-in-law Victor for his unfailing patience in helping me with computer-file transfers.

Victor is a graphic arts designer, and I especially thank him for the beautiful book cover he created. He may be reached at Victor@vrodmail.com

Many thanks, also, to my reviewers and to my husband Frank for his aid, encouragement, and patience over my piles of research.

Biblical References

Unless otherwise indicated, Bible quotations are taken from the King James Version.

Medical Disclaimer

The information in this book is for educational purposes only and should not be construed as medical advice. Readers are advised to consult competent medical professionals for their individual health and medical needs.

Although the research herein is believed to be accurate and sound, based on material available to the author, the publishers are not responsible for errors or omissions. The use or misuse of any of any information contained herein is at the sole risk and discretion of the user.

Table of Contents

1. Hidden in Plain Sight

My son, attend to my words; incline thine ear unto my sayings. . . . For they are life unto those that find them, and health to all their flesh. – Proverbs 4:20+22

"Linda brought us some peppermint tea," my husband Frank said when I came in from shopping. "I put it in the pantry."

"Great!" I said, and looked for a box of teabags while putting away my groceries. But though I searched every shelf, I couldn't spot that box of herbal tea anywhere! Finally, I gave up and called Frank to show me where he'd put it.

"It's right here," he said, pulling out a small paper bag. "I put it in front so you wouldn't miss it."

Instead of a box of teabags, Linda had brought us a brown bag of tea leaves purchased in bulk. I had overlooked the paper bag because I was looking for a colorful little box.

And that's exactly what's happened with the health secrets in the Bible. They're only "secret" because of their

1

wrappings. You see, we've been told that the *torah* — the first five books in the Bible — consist of moral rules given only to the Jews and that the New Testament contains a different set of rules for Christians.

Forgotten Meanings

When we look in a dictionary or a Bible concordance, we can find the modern meaning of any word. But many references don't go any deeper, including pocket dictionaries and *Strong's Exhaustive Concordance*. Even some lexicons don't delve into the original meaning of Hebrew words used to pen the Old Testament.

The word *torah*, which is now translated into English as the word "law," actually comes from the ancient Hebrew root *yarah*, which originally meant "to cast forth," as in sowing seed or pouring a foundation. Originally, *yarah* most often meant "sending rain," "teaching," and "instruction" (Zodhiates 1994).

Torah is a collective noun, encompassing the first five books of the Bible, and expands the meaning of the word y*arah* to mean "more rain" and "the whole of God's instruction." So, anciently, the word *torah* never meant "the law." That's a newer, man-made definition that has been added through the centuries.

Consequently, by not knowing the word's original Hebrew meaning, we believe something completely different from what the Bible writers intended! In modern lingo, the first five books of the Old Testament should really be called "teachings," rather than "the law." In fact Paul the apostle

2

sometimes referred to these books as the "oracles of God." (Romans 3:2)

False Clues and Red Herrings

Overlooking the precepts in the Old Testament, because we thought they were Jewish rules, is like missing a bag of tea leaves while looking for boxed teabags. Once we discover the true meaning of *torah* we get an entirely different picture of God, in this book often referred to as *Yahweh*. We see Him as the God of all knowledge and the One who gave us time-defying instructions on how to remain healthy and happy, rather than as a Supreme tyrant who's ready to zap us as soon as we disobey.

Many medical practitioners have understood this concept and have successfully treated disease using the Biblical principles given here. I've met people who've been healed when following these Scriptural guidelines, and I'll share their testimonies — as well as my own — in the pages that follow.

Hoarded Wealth

.

Yahweh intended the keepers of His writings to be so healthy and happy, from following His principles, that the other nations would flock to Israel to learn why it was a superior nation (Deut. 4: 5-7). When the Gentiles came to inquire, He intended the Israelites to teach them His oracles, so people from the other nations would realize that Yahweh was smarter than their man-made gods. By switching their allegiance to Yahweh and

3

following his instructions, the Gentiles could also become happy and healthy.

However, because His oracles were given specifically to them, the Israelites of old began to consider themselves better than the Gentiles. And the only Old Testament person who carried out Yahweh's desire for the Gentiles seems to be King Solomon, who rendered the Queen of Sheba speechless with his wisdom and with stories of Yahweh's greatness.

Our Most Precious Asset—Good Health

Notice in this chapter's introductory Bible verses that King Solomon declares Yahweh's words bring *health* to the flesh. In other words, they aren't meant only for spiritual guidance, but are health principles as well.

If we believe Yahweh loves us enough to sacrifice His son for us, how hard is it to believe that He wants His followers to be healthy and has openly revealed universal health principles that He Himself instituted?

If the Savior didn't want people enjoying good health, he wouldn't have spent so much time healing people and ministering to their physical needs. When we understand his remark that he and his Father are of one accord, then we start to comprehend that BOTH of them are as interested in our physical and mental well-being as they are in our eternal salvation.

You've probably read some of these Biblical health principles before and, thinking they were strictly "Jewish," may have totally ignored them as I did when I was growing up. But, as previously stated, that's like searching for teabags in a box instead of crushed leaves in a paper bag. Or, as a country-and-western song that was popular in the early 1950s goes, "I Overlooked an Orchid While Searching for a Rose."

This book presents the findings of clinical studies as well as medical research conducted at various universities, showing that Yahweh's instructions can't be surpassed as health-saving precepts. I hope readers, after examining the research, will look at Yahweh's original teachings with a new mindset and develop an appreciation of the *torah* as a vast resource on health and wellness.

Let's begin with one of the most misunderstood health principles in the Old Testament.

2. Yahweh's List

Is he the God of the Jews only? Is he not also of the Gentiles? Yes, of the Gentiles also: Seeing it is one God, which shall justify the circumcision by faith, and uncircumcision through faith. Do we then make void the law through faith? God forbid: yea, we establish the law. — Romans 3:29-31

"My son and I came over to get acquainted," I said to the mother of three little ones we'd seen playing in the yard. We'd recently moved into a new neighborhood, and my son Steve had no playmates yet.

"I made some cookies," I said, holding out the plate.

"How nice," she said, as her children gathered around and we introduced ourselves.

But as they began to help themselves, she suddenly shouted, "Wait a minute, children!"

Then she asked me if I'd made the cookies with lard. This was in the 1960s before prepared cookie dough was sold in the grocery stores.

When I assured her I'd used vegetable shortening, she gave her children permission to eat the goodies.

She invited me inside to get better acquainted while Steve stayed outdoors to play with his new friends.

"Why didn't you want them to eat anything with lard in it?" I asked.

"Lard comes from pigs, and the Bible says they're unclean," she explained, leading me into her living room.

Now I was flustered. Her husband was in my husband's Air Force squadron, and he'd assured me that these neighbors were Protestants. A Bible lay on her coffee table, yet they didn't eat pork.

"So, are you Jewish?" I asked, thinking my husband had made a mistake.

"No, we're Protestants," she answered.

"Oh," I paused, trying to remember what I'd learned in Sunday school. "I thought those rules about unclean animals were only for the Jews."

"Oh, that's not true," she assured me. "God wants *all* his children to be healthy, not just the Jewish ones!"

Then she reminded me that trichinosis can be contracted from undercooked ham, and she quoted several other Bible texts about health and our bodies, as well.

That was my introduction to the concept that Yahweh wants only the best for His children.

A Different Mindset

Growing up, I'd decided that Yahweh was an angry tyrant who dished out a lot of curses in the Old Testament and that

8

Christ came and died for us in order to appease the Father's anger. Starting over with the Gentiles, I was taught, the Savior nullified the precepts in the Old Testament.

Before I left my neighbor's house that day, I had a new picture of my heavenly Father and went home to read Leviticus Eleven more carefully.

Was it true that those laws were actually health principles and not arbitrary rules strictly for the descendants of Jacob?

I was surprised when I began studying more deeply into these things.

Bill's Carbuncles

A carbuncle is an ugly raised pimple with a hard core that requires squeezing to relieve the pressure. I squeezed a few for Bill, my first husband, and can testify that when the core is popped to release the pus, the smell is putrid.

Bill was plagued by carbuncles that erupted behind his ears every few months. Shortly after reading Leviticus 11 with a new attitude, I told Bill I didn't want to cook pork products any more since the Bible said we aren't even supposed to touch pigs' dead bodies. I suggested he satisfy his craving for pork products by eating his lunch on the military base where he worked.

About nine months later, Bill announced that he hadn't had a carbuncle in a long time, "ever since we stopped using pork," he said. I was surprised that he made the connection, because many of us don't realize how much our daily habits

9

affect our health. I was also surprised to learn that he'd personally decided not to eat pork away from home.

Bill is gone now, but he never had another carbuncle as long as he stayed away from pork products.

Half-Truths!

People who think Christ's death suddenly made unclean animals safe to eat refer to Peter's vision in Acts 10 to try to prove their claim. But they pick out a few verses to build their case and ignore the true interpretation of the event, explained by Peter himself.

The Jewish religious leaders had become extremely exclusive and considered the Gentiles to be "unclean dogs." Therefore, because Christ wanted to extend the offer of salvation to the Gentiles, he needed to show Peter and the other disciples that they should stop considering the Gentiles as "unclean" scum and dirty dogs.

Although some Bible versions claim, following this vision, that God was now pronouncing the unclean meats to be clean, that statement — usually in parentheses or written in italics — is strictly someone's personal opinion and doesn't appear in any of the original manuscripts. It also contradicts all the statements that say God is the same yesterday, today, and tomorrow.

The Bible says Peter spent some time pondering the vision because the Savior said he hadn't come to proclaim a "new" doctrine. It took Peter a little while to realize Yahweh had never called the Gentiles "unclean." Only the Jews had done so.

After prayer and his encounter with the Gentile believer Cornelius, Peter gives the REAL reason for the vision, starting in verse 19 of Acts 10, which tells the "rest of the story" and explains the vision's true interpretation.

What's the Deal?

Leviticus 11 lists the clean and unclean animals. The unclean ones fall into three categories: (1) scavengers, like vultures, pigs, and lobsters, that eat dead plants, garbage, and carrion; (2) those that act as filter feeders, like clams and oysters, whose role is to purify our rivers, lakes, and oceans; and (3) predators, like lions, snakes, and alligators, who keep down the animal population.

Seeing Is Believing

"I was walking up the road when I saw a dog inside the neighbor's pigpen," my landlady's mother told me one day when we were living in Germany.

"The dog must have eaten something that didn't agree with him because he started vomiting," she said. "And while he was still upchucking, a pig came over and started eating the vomit. After that, I stopped eating anything that comes from pigs."

"Is that right?" I asked, wondering if I'd heard her correctly.

"Yes," she continued. "Every time I see a piece of ham or bacon, I remember that filthy pig feasting on dog's vomit, and I'm not even tempted to eat any!"

This woman claimed she had never read the Bible, but she grasped one of Yahweh's health secrets, just by applying common sense to her observation. She had no desire to eat second-hand vomit.

Home on the Range

In the old West, cowboys held shooting rallies, to cut down the rattlesnake population. But, as time passed, they found a better solution. They began keeping pigs around the corral because pigs will stamp on rattlers and kill them. Snake venom doesn't seem to harm pigs (Kaneshiros 2010), which are believed to get their immunity to snake bite from their thick layer of fat. But pigs have only one sweat gland on their hoof, for eliminating poisons; so the snake venom may still be present in the fat when a piece of bacon hits the breakfast plate.

My friend Ruth says her mother grew up on a pig farm and often saw their pigs eat snakes. Her mother, who hated pork, said she'd even seen one of their pigs eat a dog.

"A dead dog," I said, hopefully.

"No, it was alive."

"Why didn't it just run away?" I asked.

"It was only a tiny puppy," Ruth explained. Apparently, it was no match for a hungry hog!

Hearing that, I can understand why her mother grew up hating pork.

Remember the SARS scare a few years ago? A group of researchers investigating SARS (severe acute respiratory syndrome) in China located the virus villain in seven different animal species, and all seven are on Yahweh's "Do Not Eat" list (Kaneshiros 2010).

Noah lived hundreds of years before Moses came on the scene. And according to Genesis 7:2 Noah already knew which animals Yahweh considered safe to eat, long before there were any Israelites. But after the flood the Egyptians worshipped frogs and other creatures, and the sons of Jacob may have forgotten some of Yahweh's original teachings during their years of Egyptian bondage. Therefore, Yahweh repeated them for all to hear when they reached Mt. Sinai.

Yahweh, a Multi-Tasking God

When Yahweh sent the plague of frogs upon the Egyptians, he was teaching at least three lessons. One was to show the Egyptians that their frog gods could be a terrible menace when out of control; the second was to show everyone that He was superior to Egypt's frog gods; and the third was to remind the sons of Jacob that He'd labeled frogs unclean. But as an additional reminder, He named all the safe and unsafe animals again, after they reached Mt. Sinai.

Too Small for the Naked Eye

A missionary doctor, who took a man for cataract surgery in France, told us what the surgeon said afterwards.

"Do you, by chance, ever eat raw frog legs?" he asked the patient.

"All the time. I love them."

"Why do you ask him that?" The missionary was curious.

"Because when we removed this man's lens, it had a parasite attached to it," the doctor explained. "It's the kind of parasite I've seen only in the eyes of people who eat raw frogs' legs, so I thought I'd ask."

This parasite, the *Gnathostoma,* is found mainly in raw or undercooked infected freshwater eels, frogs, birds, and reptiles living in tropical and subtropical areas. Although some people develop fever and other digestive disturbances after swallowing this parasite, many people have no symptoms at first. However, as the parasite matures and moves around in the body, it can cause severe health problems. As far as the eye is concerned, *Gnathostoma* has been implicated in cataract formation, glaucoma, and even retinal detachment (CDC 2012).

And that's only one kind of parasite found in animals on Yahweh's "unsafe to eat" list. Not too long ago, Florida health authorities warned Tampa Bay residents against eating frogs and giant African land snails because they carry *trifecta*, little microbes that cause meningitis. The microbes apparently come from the *Angiostronglyus Cantonenesis* parasite which frogs and snails pick up from rat droppings (Tampa Bay 2011).

The same missionary who told us about the eye parasite had served in several different temperate zones. He said he'd observed high rates of leprosy in hot climates where the people's diets were mainly wild boars and wart hogs. But in colder climates, according to him, the people who ate largely of swine developed arthritis rather than leprosy. His observation reminded me of an elderly church organist we knew.

"My father raised hogs when I was little, and we butchered our own animals," this organist told me. "I contracted trichinosis at a young age, but it wasn't diagnosed until I was much older. By then, arthritis had already set in."

She walked in a bent-over position, suffering back- and leg- pain the rest of her life; blaming her misery on arthritis. She *did* grow up in Maine, a cold climate. But arthritic pain usually lessens during the day, as the person moves around and loosens up the joints. Her pain never did; at least that's what she claimed.

After that, I did my own research to see if the missionary doctor was right. And, yes, leprosy is more prevalent in warm, tropical climates where hogs are a major part of the diet. When leprosy was rampant in Norway, the authorities there blamed it on flesh foods imported from the Dutch Indies, a warmer climate than theirs.

Leprosy's L-O-N-G Story

But leprosy isn't caused by the *trichina* worm. In the 1800s Dr. Hansen isolated the *Mycobacterium leprae*, which causes the disease; and leprosy's name has been changed, in his honor, to "Hansen's disease." Many people think leprosy has been eradicated because we never hear about it; but that's only because the name's been changed. Lepers in America are still treated at the National Hansen's Disease Program (NHDP) site in Baton Rouge, Louisiana.

Speaking of Louisiana, pathologists believe the armadillo — designated by the Creator as "unsafe for humans" — may be a leprosy carrier in our Southern states. Also, a big lawsuit in Japan in 2005 disclosed that authorities had destroyed many infants born to lepers there. It's known that many Japanese peasants consume cat- and dog- flesh, both of which are on Yahweh's "not for human consumption" list.

While the *trichina* worm burrows into human joints to cause its damage, the microbe that causes leprosy, although more deadly, has a harder time setting up housekeeping. Some kinds of bacteria can double their population in about ten minutes, but the *Mycobacterium leprae* takes much longer — up to thirteen days, actually — to replicate itself. This bacterium doesn't like human body heat but must enter a cell in order to begin reproducing. As soon as it has successfully replicated itself, it seeks a cooler location, which is why it settles just under the skin, as opposed to the *trichina* worm which can dwell in any joint or ligament (Davidson 2011).

Once a person becomes noticeably leprous, *Mycobacterium leprae* are present in all the victim's tissues and bodily secretions. But health authorities claim patients are no longer contagious after they've been treated with the modern medication that halts the disease.

If infected blood is toxic and if live *Mycobacterium leprae* can even be found in the earth where lepers' bodies have been buried, it's no wonder Yahweh called swine "not safe for humans." That could also be why He ordered His followers not even to touch a pig's cadaver. It brings glory to Him when His followers remain free from disease by obeying His statutes.

Deep, Dark Secrets

We knew a man who had delivered fresh eggs in the 1930s, and he had lots of stories to tell about his younger days. He wouldn't touch any pork products. When asked why, he told us this:

"I had yellow jaundice, and my doctor told me it was from eating pork."

We had no reason to doubt his story, since the few times we ate with him, we saw him refuse to eat anything made from, or cooked in the same dish with, pork. But how did his doctor know a person could get jaundice from eating pork products? Is it a secret that doctors reveal only when one of their patients becomes jaundiced? Why hasn't the word spread?

When I was studying home economics, I remember being cautioned to cook pork a long time, in order to kill the *trichina* worm. But nobody ever warned me about jaundice. Why not?

Not So Secret

The evening news often relates incidents of shellfish poisoning somewhere on the continent. All those critters that crawl on the ocean floor are there to eat the garbage, digest the disgusting stuff, and clean up the crud in the waters. Unfortunately, people who haven't learned Yahweh's health rules often ingest those microbes and parasites, and suffer the consequences, when they consume these filth-eating creatures.

Since the 1950s, oysters in the Chesapeake Bay have been dying out in large numbers, killed off by two different pathogenic parasites. The Shellfish Pathology Laboratory has been studying the diseases caused by these parasites, trying to restore the oyster population so these filter feeders will be able to keep our waterways free of disease once again (DEAAH 2009).

In the meantime, other diseases are affecting "mussels, cockles, clams, scallops, oysters, crabs, and lobsters" in Central America, the Pacific states, and New England (CDC 2009). People who ingest these toxic-infested shellfish begin noticing "numbness and tingling of the face, arms, and legs." Depending on the amount of toxins consumed, the numbness "may be followed by headache, dizziness, and lack of muscular coordination." The same source reports that severe cases suffer muscle paralysis and respiratory failure, ending in death anywhere from two to twenty-five hours after eating the diseased shellfish.

Governmental Confirmation

During World War II when some of our pilots were being shot down over the Pacific, military advisers asked the government to provide a list of the marine life that would be safe for downed pilots to eat when they had no rations. After an extensive, expensive study of fish and other wildlife in the ocean, the government issued a little guide for pilots. Those creatures designated safe to eat were the same ones Yahweh calls "clean" in Leviticus 11:9-12.

In the Beginning

Dr. Walter Veith, a prominent South African zoology professor, has done in-depth studies on the clean and unclean animals. He discovered that Yahweh categorized fish with fins and scales as "clean" — before our waterways became polluted — because certain fish can flush waste and toxins out of their bodies through their gills.

As long as the rivers and oceans aren't too polluted, those fish can effectively rid themselves of ingested poisons and remain fairly safe for us to eat.

They CANNOT, however, eliminate the mercury which accumulates in their bodies with each of the smaller fish they eat. This mercury remains in their bodies until we eat them or they die of mercury poisoning, whichever occurs first.

Veith has a theory about the unclean animals which, according to the Bible, ate only green vegetation when they were first created. The professor believes that after man sinned certain animals were able to adapt to a carnivorous diet without dying of toxic poisoning. Yahweh, of course, knew which these would be; so He gave that information to Noah when He commanded the boat builder to take on board seven of the "clean" animals and only two — one male and one female — of the "unclean" ones. This account is found in Genesis 7:1-10.

Like the clean fish, sharks ingest many toxins from our polluted oceans, too. But in sharks these toxins turn to urea. Somehow their bodies build up a resistance to this substance, which gets stored in their fins. When dried, shark fins are nothing more than crystallized urea, a waste product found in urine. So when we order shark-fin soup in a restaurant, thinking it's a delicacy, we're actually paying big money to eat a waste product (AD 2005).

A Healthier Alternative

Some people, especially Southerners, claim they can't enjoy their greens unless they've been cooked with a ham bone for flavoring. Those folks may find they can enjoy vegetables seasoned with smoke flavoring. Most grocery stores carry at least one brand of liquid smoke seasoning. We've found it for ninety-nine cents on the same shelf with the dressings and marinades. Just add a drop or two to the water in the pot before cooking the greens, and you may be pleasantly surprised.

Some health food stores also carry bacon-flavored yeast flakes, an additional source of Vitamin B. But these flakes are more expensive than the bottled flavoring, and the liquid works just as well.

We recently learned another way to add healthful fat and flavor to our bean pot, and that is to cook cut-up eggplant in with the beans.

Higher than the Highest Thought

Because Yahweh is so much smarter than we are and is able to multi-task, He's able to teach more than one concept at a time. And since we humans consist of three entities — our minds, our physical bodies, and our spiritual natures — why wouldn't His teachings impart health to all three areas of our lives?

Though early church leaders claimed the *torah* was the method by which the Old Testament Jews were "saved" and doesn't apply to Gentiles, this chapter's introductory Bible verse reminds us that both Jews and Gentiles alike were always *saved by faith*, not by their works.

In their eagerness to make Christianity as unlike Judaism as possible, misguided religious leaders claimed the Savior's death abolished the *torah*. In doing so, they completely overlooked Yahweh's all-encompassing health principles.

If we read the New Testament carefully, we learn that it wasn't Yahweh's <u>oracles</u> in the Old Testament that the Savior criticized. It was the man-made rules and rituals the over-zealous religious leaders had added to His statutes after their return from Babylonian captivity. Many of these man-made laws conflicted with Yahweh's *torah*.

Let's look at one specific rite which second-century rabbis introduced, while trying to improve on Yahweh's original command.

3. A Cut Above

And he that is eight days old shall be circumcised among you, every man child in your generations.
— Genesis 17:12

S ince Yahweh commanded Abraham to circumcise Isaac on the "eighth day" (Gen. 17:10-14), and since the Savior was circumcised on his eighth day of life (Luke 2:21), the Kaneshiros wanted to follow the Biblical example and have their newborn son circumcised when he was eight days old too. They chose to give birth to their baby at home and located a pediatrician who agreed to come and circumcise their son when he was eight days old.

The pediatrician arrived at the appointed time, prepared to give the baby a Vitamin K shot. She said it was "standard hospital procedure" when circumcising newborns. The Kaneshiros asked her to withhold the shot, saying they had faith that Yahweh would protect their child since they were following His instructions as best they could.

The physician suggested a compromise: "All right, I'll withhold the shot before the procedure," she said. "But I'll have to stay and watch the baby awhile to make sure his blood clots. If it doesn't, I'll have to administer the Vitamin K shot so he doesn't bleed to death."

Husband and wife agreed. The pediatrician circumcised their son and stood watch, ready to give the shot. But there was no need; the baby's blood clotted just fine (Kaneshiros 2010).

Does Yahweh Care?

In their studies the Kaneshiros learned that newborn infants' blood has almost no Vitamin K, which regulates the clotting agent *prothrombin*. After five to seven days of breast feeding, the clotting agent is built up in the infant's blood. They discovered that *prothrombin's* count reaches 108 on the eighth day, the highest it ever gets. After that, it drops down to 100 where it more or less stabilizes.

The Kaneshiros' discovery agrees completely with McMillen's research (1967), which found that an eight-day-old infant has "more available *prothrombin* than on any other day of its life."

In Abraham's day, long before clamps were designed to seal off the blood vessels, who else but Yahweh could have known the safest time to circumcise a baby with the least amount of danger from hemorrhaging?

However, the type of circumcision practiced today can be dangerous to some infants, especially if they are hemophilic [bleeders]. In fact, the *Talmud* (traditions of the rabbis) "explicitly instructs that a boy must not be circumcised if he had two brothers who died due to complications arising from their circumcisions" (JE 1901). Actually, the procedure Yahweh commanded wasn't as drastic as the one performed by physicians today. Around 154 A.D. the rabbis weren't satisfied with the Biblical method and came up with one of their own. But before we investigate that switch, let's look at the history of circumcision in America.

Early Twentieth Century

"Look at this!" exclaimed the Chief of Staff at Mt. Sinai Hospital in New York.

The other doctors gathered around him, wondering what was so interesting about the patient files he'd been studying.

"Every one of these patients with cervical cancer is married to a non-Jewish man."

"So?"

"We have plenty of female patients married to Jewish men," he explained. "But they're always in here for some *other* treatment. None of them has been treated for, or even diagnosed with, cervical cancer!"

"Just a coincidence," said one.

"I think it's their diet," said another. "They don't eat pork and shellfish, you know."

"That's probably the reason," the majority agreed.

That was in the early 1900s. Word traveled to Bellevue hospital where someone searched through its records and found the same situation. According to McMillen (1967), "in 1949 gynecologists at the Mayo Clinic noted that in 568 consecutive cases of cervical cancer, not a single Jewess was among the victims." By 1954 when cervical cancer was on the increase, doctors in Boston had learned that non-Jewish women were eight-and-a-half times more likely to develop this type of cancer than those married to Jewish men.

Those physicians concluded that circumcision was the reason for the healthy cervixes of these wives. The husbands of these non-cancerous women lacked a foreskin under which bacteria can accumulate and infections can develop (Hawker 2010).

And it's true that viruses can multiply under men's foreskin — particularly the viruses that cause genital warts and cervical cancer — especially if men don't follow strict principles of personal hygiene. In fact circumcised males were considered "cleaner" than other men in ancient Egypt. One engraving in their artwork, dating back to about 2000 B.C., shows a fully-grown, standing male being circumcised. But both circumcised and uncircumcised men appear together naked in some other engravings, so it's thought that the procedure was practiced mostly as a status symbol among Egypt's upper class at that time.

Medical Progression

In 1914 Abraham Wolbarst pushed for universal circumcision in *Journal of the American Medical Association.* He wrote (Wolbarst 1914) that "the vast preponderance of modern scientific opinion on the subject is strongly in favor of circumcision as a sanitary measure and as a prophylactic against infection with venereal disease."

He was later joined by physicians like those who'd noticed that cervical cancer rates were lower among wives of circumcised men. The medical establishment in India and Great Britain followed suit, and circumcision of infants became the standard operating procedure in many hospitals.

Faulty Assumptions

In fact, because they once believed that all diseases were transmitted the same way, many doctors were certain that circumcision would end the spreading of all viruses. Eventually some even incorrectly assumed that circumcision would reduce the rates of "alcoholism, epilepsy, asthma, gout, rheumatism, curvature of the spine and headache ..... paralysis, malnutrition, night terrors, and clubfoot; eczema, convulsions and mental retardation; promiscuity, syphilis," among others (Miller 2002).

They had jumped to conclusions about the causes of all diseases. And so physicians began circumcising male babies the "Jewish" way.

But they also jumped to conclusions about the procedure. Most doctors didn't realize that the *Jewish* method of circumcising *isn't even the Biblical way*! Long before the 1900s, the Scriptural method of circumcision had done a disappearing act.

Actually, there are several kinds of circumcision; but only one of them is Biblical.

Not Yahweh's Way!

In some closed societies, adolescent males undergo circumcision to prove their manhood. This cultic rite is performed without anesthesia; and a youth wishing to prove his manhood must not cry out or show any signs of physical pain during the procedure. This cultic ritual may have been carried out in Egypt at the time of Abraham.

What Did Yahweh Really Command?

Many parents of newborns complain that circumcision is radical and unnecessary. And, as mentioned earlier, the procedure which is performed today can be hazardous to hemophiliacs (bleeders). Would a loving creator order a life-threatening procedure for male children? Not at all! There's more to the story.

The command given to Abraham was *muwl* (in *Strong's* Concordance) or *milah,* as some pronounce it, meaning "to shorten." Either way it's pronounced, the original Hebrew word meant only "cutting off the tip or the end." This command denoted a minor cutting in which only the foreskin "that extended beyond the glans" was removed. For this reason the prejudiced Romans, in ridiculing the Jews, applied the term *curtus*, meaning "cut short" to circumcised men (Horace).

Intentional Cover-Up

The ancient Greeks believed that the male body was beautiful and shouldn't be tampered with. Therefore, they considered a circumcised penis "desecrated." Like the Romans, they were also prejudiced against the Jews. So Jews were prohibited from competing in Greek and Roman sporting events which were performed naked.

But some athletic, sports-loving Jews found ways to look uncircumcised. Enough foreskin remained on Jewish males after *milah* circumcision so they could nearly reverse the procedure and appear to be uncircumcised. One popular method consisted of attaching a copper weight, called *Judeum pondum*, to the "remnant of the circumcised foreskin until, in time, [the skin] became sufficiently stretched to cover the glans" (Rubin 1980). Thus, a man could appear to have a normal penis, and not be accounted Jewish, making him eligible to compete in the games.

Such lengthening of the foreskin could not have been practiced if radical circumcision, as we know it today, was the norm back then.

Rabbinical Indignation

This practice of reversing one's circumcision angered some of the leading rabbis, who claimed those athletic Jews were denying their covenant with Abraham. So those rabbis invented a more radical procedure called *Brit Peri'ah*, which entails cutting the foreskin all the way "back to the ridge behind the glans penis" (Peron 2000). This newer procedure dates back to the second century A.D. and is NOT the method used during Christ's lifetime.

Later the religious leaders added this radical procedure to the *Talmud*, which consists of many non-Biblical Jewish traditions. And to prevent any more cover-ups, *Brit Peri'ah* was made a Jewish religious requirement.

Brit Peri'ah is the method of circumcision performed in our hospitals today. But it's NOT Biblical because it's not the type of circumcision Yahweh prescribed!

Is It Worth It?

Even though not Biblical, *radical* circumcision offers some benefits. Circumcised infants are less likely to contract a urinary tract infection (UTI) in the first year of life. The rate is

1/1000 for circumcised infants, but 1/100 for uncircumcised ones (Halta 2009).

Also, as stated earlier, wives of circumcised husbands are twenty percent less likely to develop cervical cancer (Hawker 2010). In 2007 — the most recent year numbers are available — "12,280 American women were diagnosed with cervical cancer," and 4,021 died from it (US 2010).

Recent studies in India also show that, while cervical cancer is widespread among Hindu and Christian women there, Muslim wives — whose husbands are always circumcised — rarely contract the disease.

In addition, the rate of genital warts is less in circumcised males and their female partners (Kaneshiros 2010), but poor hygiene is also considered a risk factor.

Among older adult males, penile cancer affects more uncircumcised men than others, although cigarette smoking may add to the risk.

That leaves only one physical ailment that NEVER happens to circumcised males — that of *phimosis*, a painfully rigid, too-tight foreskin.

To Be or Not to Be?

When Sammy, who hadn't been circumcised at birth, developed *phimosis* with severe pain, the doctors recommended circumcision. The five-year-old spent one night in the hospital, and circumcision solved his problem. Adolescent boys and young men may also develop this condition.

But not every uncircumcised male develops *phimosis*, and — for those who do — there's a pharmaceutical cream which may soften the skin somewhat.

Many males who deal with the problem for any length of time, though, often undergo circumcision as a last resort. According to the Men's Health website most men who've suffered with *phimosis* report a positive healing experience and a wish that they'd been circumcised sooner (Men's Health 2009).

Although "urologists who deal with the problems of uncircumcised men cannot understand why all newborns are not circumcised," (Schoen 1993) medical researchers no longer believe circumcision is the cure-all it was once hailed to be. For that reason, and also because many parents have complained about the harsh, non-Biblical procedure practiced today, Medicaid funding has been cut for routine infant circumcision.

Just for the Record

The ONLY cancer rate that circumcision has been proven to lower is cervical cancer in women. Yet some health officials have erroneously claimed that circumcision prevents prostate cancer in men as well. That claim isn't true, since prostate cancer isn't "caught," as we'll see in Chapter Four.

In addition, some have pressured men to become circumcised as a preventative for HIV. But not all viruses lurk under the foreskin. Dentists wear face masks when working on patients because, as we've been warned, HIV may be transmitted through sneezing, coughing, and saliva as well as the bodily fluids secreted during sexual intercourse.

Be assured: Circumcision is NOT a preventative for HIV and the majority of STDs (sexually transmitted diseases); but Yahweh has given several sexual guidelines that definitely relate to people's health.

Health Risks for Heterosexuals

Everyone who has read much on the subject knows that STDs are more prevalent among the sexually active population than among those who believe in abstaining from sexual intercourse outside marriage. But here are additional recent discoveries from medical journals:

One study found that women who receive anal sex "are at a higher risk for contracting anal cancer" than women who don't (IDN 1997).

Health Risks for Homosexuals

Most homosexual females face a "significantly higher risk of bacterial vaginosis, breast cancer and ovarian cancer" than do heterosexual women (MISH 1999).

Males receiving anal sex have a 4,000 percent increased risk of developing anal cancer (BTL 2000), and nearly half of the 20-year-old men currently receiving it "will not reach their 65th birthday" (IJE 2009).

After reviewing the medical literature, some of us may want to rethink our position on the verses found in Leviticus 20:13, 15, and 25. Instead of viewing these statutes as rules to keep us from "doing our own thing," why not see them as principles that — if followed — will ensure our health and happiness?

Now let's look at some cancers which are NOT transmitted from person to person.

4. The China Study

*That all the people of the earth may know that
the Lord is God, and that there is none else.*
— First Kings 8:60

M any people blame chemicals and pollutants for cancerous
tumors. And it's true that breast cancer is quite prevalent
in the little town where I grew up, just down-river from
Monsanto® chemical plant. But not everybody in the town gets
cancer.

Not Just Air Pollutants?

Research shows that our bodies are bombarded by
chemicals and pollutants every day. In fact, the authorities say
every one of us has jet fuel in our blood samples. But not
everyone gets cancerous tumors. Researchers have discovered
that something must happen to these toxic agents in our bodies
before they turn cancerous. These foreign agents, called *foci,* can
lie dormant in our bodies for years. Studies show they become

cancerous only when attacked by certain amino acids (Campbell 2006).

The China Study, the most comprehensive cancer study conducted so far, revealed that certain cancers are more prevalent in affluent areas of China. The Campbells, who conducted the study, observed the eating habits of those people and found that as families grew wealthy they tended to eat a richer diet, while poorer families tended to eat home-grown vegetables and fewer delicacies.

After comparing the diets of people with high and low cancer rates, the Campbells discovered that the people who got cancer of the breast, prostate, or colon ate large amounts of animal protein (meat or dairy products). But in the groups with low rates of cancer, the people's diets contained very small amounts of animal flesh and dairy foods.

The First Tests

The Campbells brought the results of their study back to America and tested their hypothesis in the laboratory. First they injected all the rats with *aflotoxin*, a known cancer-causing bacteria. They gave one set of rats a diet containing at least 20 percent animal protein; the control group received none. As the Campbells had hypothesized, all the rats in the 20 percent animal-protein group developed cancerous tumors; while those in the control group didn't.

Since then, other researchers have duplicated the Campbell's study and caused laboratory animals to develop cancerous tumors by feeding them a diet containing at least 20 percent meat or dairy products. In another experiment, animals remained cancer-free on a diet containing less than 5 percent animal protein. Although the Campbells used dairy protein in their study, it didn't seem to matter whether the animal protein was from meat or dairy products — the results were the same (Campbell 2006).

Stimulating Stuff

Food chemists agree that red meat and butter are stimulants, but such news somehow never reaches the general public. I wonder why? Could it be that the media is controlled by certain lobbyists? Hmmm.

My father loved meat! Any kind was okay, but he chose rare steak, with the blood still oozing out, as often as he could. He developed cancer in his late 60s and had his prostate surgically removed.

Dad tried giving up meat several times. But he mistook the headache and tired feeling, which are actually withdrawal symptoms, for a sign that he wasn't getting enough protein and went back to eating meat each time. A few years later, the disease returned as bone cancer in his shoulder. He had that cut out, too, but it finally spread to his lungs, and he spent his last year on oxygen.

Dad's diet was heavy on animal protein. The Campbells would have loved doing a study on him!

They'd have loved doing a study on Mauve, too, a distant relative. She developed breast cancer in her late fifties. The cancer spread first to her back and hips and, finally, to her brain. Her husband was a gourmet cook, and they ate a very rich diet with expensive cuts of meat.

Both were heavy smokers, but Mauve quit the habit when she was first diagnosed with cancer. She began drinking more milk, thinking it would help build her stamina. She didn't cut back on meat, though, and her husband continued cooking rich, exotic dishes. Between the second-hand smoke and the high animal protein intake, the Campbells would say it's no surprise that her cancer metastasized.

The China Study aside, other researchers have found the same results. Take the following inventory of your eating habits, and check your answers with the recent research:

(1) I drink _____ glasses of milk each day.

(2) I eat _____ eggs at least once a day.

(3) I eat butter or cheese at least _____ times a day.

(4) I eat meat at least _____ times in a day.

Here's the cancer risk for each of the items numbered above:

(1) "The Iowa Women's Health Study found that women who consumed more than one glass of milk per day had a 73 percent greater chance of ovarian cancer than women who drank less than one glass per day" (Physicians 2007).

(2) Daily users of eggs have 2.8 times greater risk of cancer "than those who limit eggs to once a week" (Douglass 1998).

(3) Butter and cheese users have "2-3 times greater risk of breast cancer" than non-consumers (Douglass 1998).

(4) Breast cancer is "3.8 times greater in people consuming meat daily compared to vegetarians" (Douglass 1998). "Nutritional factors, especially meat, fat, and dairy intake, have been linked to greater risk of [prostate] disease" (Chan 1998).

(3+4) "Suggestive positive associations were also seen between fatal prostate cancer and the consumption of milk, cheese, eggs, and meat" (Snowden 1984). And a more detailed study found that "positive correlation between foods and cancer mortality rates were particularly strong in the case of meats and milk for breast cancer; milk for prostate and ovarian cancer; and meats for colon cancer" (Rose 1986).

PSA Factors

Dean Ornish, M.D., studied 97 male patients with high PSA levels (early-stage prostate cancer) and put half of them on a low-fat vegan diet. (Vegan meals contain no flesh foods or animal byproducts.) Those patients' PSA levels dropped by 4 percent that first year. People in the control group – who were given no special diet – saw no drop in their PSA levels. And, in fact, six of them required surgery before the year ended because their PSA levels rose to a dangerously high level, as do all those males who succumb to prostate cancer (Campbell 2006).

Many males, whose fathers also had prostate cancer, get the dreaded disease because they've followed the same lifestyle as their fathers, including their diets, and make no changes after they've been diagnosed as *precancerous*: that is, showing a higher-than-normal PSA count.

A UCLA study (SH 2003) found that men's blood serum shows "demonstrable cancer-inhibiting power within as little as eleven days after beginning a low-fat diet and exercise regimen." Animal products are not considered "low-fat" since the leanest chicken available today consists of 27 percent fat, and the leanest beef sold commercially contains 55 percent fat.

By the way, there have been at least 23 different research projects on the role of animal protein in prostate cancers. And every one of them found a positive correlation (Hope-2 2011).

Long Ago and Far Away

The first time I ever heard of anyone's not eating meat was back in the early 1950s when Linda joined my tap-dancing class. She told everyone that her father worked in a meat-packing business and never ate meat. In fact, he ordered his wife never to cook meat for any of his meals and never to put cold cuts in his lunch. After working with it all day and knowing how it was processed, he developed an aversion to meat products.

At the time, the Genesis account of Yahweh's original diet for mankind had never impressed me, though I'd read it a number of times. By the time I took the text seriously, my immune system had become compromised after years of strenuous dancing and pushing myself too hard. When I switched to a vegetarian diet and gave up white bread, my health began improving.

Linda's meatless father had completely slipped my mind until my parents worried about my switch to vegetarianism. But thanks to Linda's testimony, I just reminded them that her father lived to a ripe old age.

Priscilla

One of the saddest cases I've ever known concerns Priscilla, a friend of a friend. My friend — Priscilla's best friend — had read the warnings about meat's connection with breast cancer and shared some health literature with Priscilla. But Priscilla believed the myth, that you couldn't get enough protein from a plant diet; and she loved meat and cheese. Besides, she'd asked her family physician, and he assured her that cancer was in no way connected to anyone's diet.

Priscilla had already undergone two mastectomies before we were introduced at a vegetarian buffet. Servings on her plate included macaroni and cheese, potato-and-egg salad, sweet potato pudding (containing more egg), and spinach casserole made with more eggs and cheese.

When I learned — a few months later — that she'd developed cancer of the esophagus, I was trying to think of a tactful way to tell her about *The China Study*; but her best friend stopped me.

"I've already tried warning her," the friend assured me. "You won't get anywhere. Priscilla just loves her meat! Besides, her doctor told her it was good for her."

Several times I heard Priscilla brag about being a cancer survivor. But her recovery wasn't complete. About a year after her esophagus surgery, the cancer had metastasized to her lungs. This time it was terminal.

She was bedridden for several months and existed on morphine until death finally claimed her.

Prophets without Profit

It's lonely being the only prophet around, especially when the truths you want to share aren't popular, so I was delighted to learn that two local physicians have switched to vegan diets, enjoy increased health and vigor, and currently advocate vegetarianism for many of their ailing patients. It was reported in our *Richmond Times-Dispatch*, and the article was archived on the internet (Times 2010).

That particular news item probably didn't make headlines all over America, but maybe former president Bill Clinton's testimony did. After his heart surgery, he read that stents don't reverse any of the damage to a person's arteries, so he went on a vegan diet partly to please his daughter Chelsea and partly to see if it would improve his condition. In a 2010 television interview he reported that he not only felt better in time for Chelsea's wedding, but he also dropped back to his high school weight. He said his health has improved so much that he intends to continue a meatless lifestyle.

Addiction Depiction

The Campbells reported, "Dairy intake is one of the most consistent dietary predictors for prostate cancer in the published literature" (Campbell 2006). Too bad my father wasn't alive when their book came out. Dad's favorite between-meal snacks were salted popcorn in a bowl of milk or, if he couldn't find any cheese slices to go with his crackers, crushed soda crackers in milk. Actually, cheese is hard to give up if you're addicted to it. Dad's favorite dessert was the piece of cheese that went with his apple pie.

I know how addictive cheese can be. When Frank and I decided to stop eating animal byproducts, it was easy to stop bringing cheese home from the grocery store. But we both occasionally hankered for pizza while going through withdrawal. People who claim cheese *isn't* addictive should try giving it up! Maybe they'll be like Samuel Clemens, who claimed he could give up smoking any time he wanted to. After all, he'd done it many times!

As far back as 1994, the American Cancer Society knew that "breast cancer rates are lower in populations that consume plant-based diets," but many of us believe that statistics apply only to the other fellow — until we actually become ill. Even then, we like to blame our illness on fate or pollution. Some people even blame God! These folks ignore the facts that "we are what we eat," and it's possible "to dig our graves with our teeth."

No Meat?!!!

The Bible tells the story of Daniel the prophet, who was taken captive and brought to Babylon when Jerusalem was destroyed by Nebuchadnezzar. The king gave orders that the smartest and healthiest captives should live in the palace, eat the same food as the royal family, and be taught by the nation's wise men and magicians.

Daniel 1:8 says, "But Daniel purposed in his heart that he would not defile himself with the portion of the king's meat nor with the wine which he drank." For this reason Daniel approached the prince of eunuchs, in whose charge he and his friends had been placed, and requested a plain, simple vegetarian diet of *pulse*. The man agreed to serve Daniel and his three friends (who were later thrown into the fiery furnace) plain vegetables for ten days, after which they would be examined for weakness, illness, or mental defects.

At the end of the ten-day period, Daniel and his friends were found to be not only healthier, but also ten times wiser, than all the other students in the king's academy. For that reason, they were allowed to continue on their diet of *pulse*. The entire story is in the first couple chapters of the Book of Daniel.

According to ancient historian Josephus, *pulse* means "sprouted seeds." And, according to Dr. Paulien, "Wheat, mung beans, alfalfa seeds, and soy beans make excellent sprouts," increasing "the nutritional value of these seeds tremendously by creating new vitamins" (Iglesias 1998).

Preparing meals without adding meats for flavor can be a new experience, but the health benefits are worth it. The easiest way to get started is to have brown rice and beans three times a week with a big salad.

For variety, you can learn to sprout beans yourself (saves money), steam them lightly, and add them to a salad. There are enough kinds of beans to get a good variety every week.

Check your local library for vegan cookbooks with directions for sprouting beans, nuts, and seeds so you can be as healthy and wise as the prophet Daniel was.

In summary, the results of many independent researchers and University studies, like the findings of the Cancer project and *The China Study*, show that Yahweh's original vegetarian diet — as stated in Genesis 1:29 — is the most healthful one for humans.

Flesh foods were introduced only later, under extenuating circumstances.

5. Manly Men

Lo, this only have I found, that God hath made man upright; but they have sought out many inventions. — Ecclesiastes 7:29

We were at a bridal shower, and I was sitting near a man whose wife was helping with the gifts. Cake, ice cream, and punch were the main refreshments.

"I can't wait to get home and eat some man's food," the man said.

"What's that?" I asked. "Chips and dip?"

"No," he said, patting his stomach. "Beefsteak. That's MAN food!"

What Makes Men Manly?

His statement reminded me of some research I'd come across about men's hormones. Testosterone is the hormone that makes men feel and act masculine. A British study measured testosterone levels in 696 Oxford University men, of which 233 were vegan (ate no animal products), 237 were vegetarian (consumed milk and dairy products but no meat), and 237 ate meat most days of the week. The tests showed (British 2000) that "vegans had higher testosterone levels than vegetarians and meat eaters."

Breast cancer is becoming more prevalent among men, who often suffer a decrease in testosterone as they age. Overweight men are apparently getting too much estrogen, which is found in cow's milk, cheese, ice cream, and beef, and which — according to Dr. Horton — attacks the *foci*, the carcinogenic agents mentioned in Chapter Four, and turns them into cancer cells (Horton 2007).

If estrogen destroys testosterone in men, then is red meat really "masculine" food? Keith Akers, a historian who researched documents from the papal archives, may disagree.

James, the Brother of Jesus

According to Akers, ancient documents portray Christ's original apostles as vegetarians (Akers 2000). The list includes James, Christ's brother, who headed the first council of believers in Jerusalem as mentioned in the Book of Acts. It stands to reason that, if *they* were all vegetarians, then the Messiah must certainly have been a vegetarian as well. After all, they claimed to be his followers.

It's true, there are several Biblical accounts of the Savior's feeding the crowds loaves and fishes. But there are two possible explanations. The first is that some historians believe

Roman church leaders may have added the fish tales to the Bible in later years when they set aside Friday as "fish day" to boost the languishing fishing industry.

Another reasonable explanation is that the historians who reported on early Christian groups may have believed — as some do today — that vegetarians eat white meat. In fact, when people learn I'm a vegetarian, some often ask, "But you eat fish, right?" So some historians back then may have thought the same way. A real vegetarian knows that fish and chicken aren't vegetables.

The Messiah's disciples would naturally want to emulate him and follow his example. Therefore, we can conclude that, if His disciples ate no meat — at least no RED meat, Christ must also have been a vegetarian. But the Savior was no sissy. So much for MAN food!

Early Followers of the Savior

Before the early Christian congregations came under the auspices of the Roman church, there were many isolated groups of Jewish-believers in Christ – as well as Gentile converts -- who refused to eat the flesh of animals. They copied the diet eaten by the disciples and early church fathers, believing that we shouldn't kill animals merely to gratify our appetites. And through the years, many deep thinkers have felt the same way.

An internet search will provide a lengthy list of vegetarians who were well known in their day. One of these was George Bernard Shaw, who in the 1940s said, "We are the living graves of murdered beasts, slaughtered to satisfy our appetites."

And God said, Behold, I have given you every herb bearing seed, which is upon the face of all the earth, and every tree, in the which is the fruit of a tree yielding seed; to you it shall be for meat.
— Genesis 1:29

Because Yahweh permitted meat eating after the flood, some religious teachers claim He *added* meat eating to the Genesis diet.

The idea that Yahweh would change His mind after giving us the ideal diet is wishful thinking. Common sense tells us that, since there was no vegetation after the flood, He would instruct Noah and his family which creatures could be safely eaten [clean versus unclean] until the earth's vegetation had time to replenish itself (Gen. 7:2).

Just because Yahweh repeated the list for the multitudes coming out of Egypt is no reason to think that He was now upgrading His original instructions. After all, He said He never changes the words that have come from His mouth (Psalm 89:34). Yahweh wants His followers to be disease free, yet He never forces us to obey. He says, "Believe and live." But we make our own choices, and some of us are eating our way to illness and an early grave.

The Inside Scoop

The teeth of carnivorous animals are all sharp and pointed, and their jaws move only up and down, for biting and tearing, while we humans have molars, for crushing and grinding, and jaws that move sideways for more grinding.

In addition, carnivores' digestive systems are designed differently than those of herbivores. Their intestines are much shorter, for quick expulsion of waste; and their livers contain large amounts of *uricase*, an enzyme that helps break down uric acid. We humans, on the other hand, don't produce *uricase*, which may be one reason that heavy meat-eaters get gout, a painful ailment caused by excess uric acid in the system. In addition, our intestines are "designed to retain solids in them until all beneficial nutrients are extracted," and have entered the blood stream (Diamond 1985).

A more recent study shows that waste products take 72 hours to be eliminated from the colon of meat-eating humans and partial vegetarians (who consume eggs and dairy products), while the feces of raw foodists and vegans are eliminated from the body in about 24 hours.

Waste products ferment in the body due to a lack of fiber needed to push them through the colon in a timely manner (WCRF 1997). The results are flatulence, intestinal problems, polyps in the colon, and accumulation of excess fat cells, to name a few.

Barbecued Fibs

When I became a vegetarian in 1962, I started eating more cheese because, like many others, I believed that vegetarians had to get their protein from dairy products. That myth is largely promoted by the dairy industry and has been proven false by the China Study, the Cancer Project, and other reliable research.

Most nutritionists claim the only way a person can develop a protein deficiency is if s/he is also suffering from malnutrition. This occurs mostly in countries where there's a famine. "The protruding bellies of the starving children in famine-stricken countries indicate a protein deficiency" (Hope-1 2010).

The majority of menus offered in fast-food restaurants consist of fried foods and refined breads and, except for the salads, contain few nutrients. Interestingly, nutritionists claim that people who eat an abundance of processed foods are more at risk for a protein deficiency than those who eat plenty of raw fruits and crunchy vegetables.

In all my years as a vegetarian, I've never met anyone who was diagnosed with a protein deficiency. I've met a few who had B-12 deficiencies, though. A vegetarian friend of mine ate an abundance of dairy products for years, to make up for not eating meat, yet she has to go for Vitamin B-12 shots every month.

Who says you must take Vitamin B-12 supplements if you give up meat and dairy products? Many reliable sources claim that one milligram of Vitamin B-12 will last a person over two years, and healthy individuals usually carry around a five-year supply in their bodies.

Since our intestines weren't designed to handle flesh foods, meat often putrefies before it is thoroughly digested. This putrefaction hampers the secretion of the "intrinsic factor" in the stomach and retards the production of B-12, which is made in the body. So flesh eaters are more apt to develop a Vitamin B-12 deficiency than vegetarians are (Diamond 1985).

Verifying the Diamonds' claim, *the American Journal of Clinical Nutrition* carried an article by Victor Herbert stating that B-12 is "recycled from liver bile . . . reabsorbed in an efficient way for the body's homeostasis and prevents adult vegans from developing B-12 deficiencies" (AJCN 1996).

The above studies refer to adult vegans. Apparently some babies are born with a faulty system for regulating B-12 in their bodies. These infants will need B-12 injections, regardless of their diets.

Another Myth Debunked

The truth about B-12 was known as far back as 1959, but the myth is still being propagated — mostly by those who can make a profit by scaring people into buying their product. Any lie that's spread long enough becomes part of the culture and is accepted even by intelligent people who don't take the time to study the subject more deeply.

Part of the dietary myth is that if we leave off dairy products, we must take Vitamin B-12 supplements because it isn't found in plant food. So when I saw a bottle of supplements labeled "vegetarian formula," I emailed the company to ask the

53

source of their supplement. They responded that their vegetarian Vitamin B-12 was from molasses. If B-12 doesn't exist in plant food, how can it be extracted from molasses, which comes from plants? It takes only a little common sense to realize we've been lied to by profiteers.

I'm not saying people should *never* take B-12 supplements! Those who hate green vegetables and eat an abundance of processed foods might need them, especially if they are sickly and a health professional says they're deficient in the vitamin. In fact, several people thought to have Alzheimer's disease actually recovered when their B-12 levels were increased.

The truth is, the only vegans or vegetarians who will suffer a Vitamin B-12 deficiency are those who (1) already had a faulty intrinsic factor when they became vegetarians, or (2) fill up on processed foods lacking the essential B vitamins, or (3) get too much sugar in their diets, thus destroying the B vitamins in their bodies. As my high school English teacher used to say, "A word to the wise is sufficient."

The short story is that all segments of the population, including meat eaters, can develop Vitamin B-12 deficiencies if they eat mostly desserts, junk foods, and highly processed concoctions.

One medical researcher has claimed, though, that a blood sample isn't the best indicator of a person's real B-12 count. It seems that the amount of B-12 found in a woman's vaginal fluid and a man's semen is seven to ten times greater than the amount found in their blood samples.

Too Close for Comfort

Check the following statements that describe your habits:

1. Cold-cut sandwiches or a grinder daily   _____
2. Skinless chicken about 5 times a week   _____
3. Pork products twice a week   _____
4. Meat at least once a day   _____
5. Meat *fewer than* five times a week   _____

Compare your answers with the following research:

(1) The World Cancer Research Fund, after a review of more than 7,000 clinical studies, linked "processed meats such as bacon, ham, salami, corned beef and some sausages . . . to a high risk of bowel cancer" (WCRF 1997).

(2) Some people switch from red meat to chicken and remove the skin, which is known to be very fatty. But a Harvard Medical School study of bladder cancer, published in 2010, reported that even those who ate skinless chicken five times a week had a "52 percent greater risk of getting bladder cancer" than those who seldom ate chicken (Hope-2 2011).

(3) Other studies (WCRF 1997) have "singled out beef and pork consumption and have concluded there is a higher risk for pancreatic cancer with a higher intake of these foods."

(4) A Japanese study found that "people consuming meat daily had higher death rates from kidney cancer than those eating

meat less frequently." Also, Harvard studies (Barnard and Howard 1995) showed that "daily meat eaters have approximately three times the colon cancer risk" of those who rarely eat meat.

(5) Twentieth-century Germany- and England-based studies (Thorogood et al 1994) showed "that vegetarians were about 40 percent less likely to develop cancer compared to meat eaters."

Female Figures

Several studies have found four factors contributing to breast cancer in women:

(1) starting menstrual periods at a young age,

(2) entering menopause at a late age,

(3) high levels of estrogen in the blood,

(4) high blood cholesterol.

Interestingly enough, the four preceding factors can all be affected by our diets:

(1) Cow's milk has been linked to young girls' maturing too early;

(2) Lack of dietary fiber has been linked to late menopause;

(3) Excess animal protein raises the estrogen level;

(4) Only mushrooms, flesh foods and animal byproducts are sources of dietary cholesterol. (I've misplaced my original

source concerning mushrooms, which some call *vegetables*, although they're actually fungi.)

Our bodies naturally produce about 300 mg., a sufficient amount, of HDL cholesterol each day. This GOOD cholesterol lodges just under our skin so it can convert sunlight into the Vitamin D our bodies need (Gominak 2011). HDL also helps clean our arteries.

LDL cholesterol, also called *dietary cholesterol*, comes from the foods we eat and is the BAD guy. When we eat cholesterol-laden foods, we place an extra burden on our liver and kidneys. Clogged arteries contribute to high blood pressure, strokes, and heart attacks.

[Author's note, (2018 edition): Several recent studies show that high cholesterol is no longer considered a valid indicator of an ensuing heart attack. In fact, when my husband had his heart attack, his cholesterol was fine; it was his triglycerides that were abnormally high.]

Pass the Buck, Please

Some people will refuse to believe any research or statistics connecting cancer's link to people's lifestyle. They blame pollutants, asbestos, and fate. Pollutants truly *are* carcinogenic agents. But the Associated Press recently reported the results of a study showing that the majority of cancers are directly related to one's lifestyle (AP 2010).

BBC news recently reported that only "one in 25 cancers is linked to a person's job," such as being exposed to chemicals or asbestos.

Here are recent statistics about men and women's cancers:

"In men, 6.9% (9,600) of cancer cases were linked to a lack of fruit and vegetables, 4.9% (7,800) to occupation, 4.6% (7,300) to alcohol, 4.1% (6,500) to overweight and obesity and 3.5% (5,500) to excessive sun exposure and sunbeds."

"In women, 6.9% (10,800) were linked to overweight and obesity, 3.7% (5,800) to infections such as HPV [the human papilloma virus that causes cervical cancer], 3.6% (5,600) to excessive sun exposure and sunbeds, 3.4% (5,300) to lack of fruit and vegetables and 3.3% (5,100) to alcohol" (BBC 2011).

As noted above, only 3.7% of the women's cancers were linked to infections or viruses; and only 4.9% of men's cancers were related to their occupations; the rest were all lifestyle related.

The above findings agree with those of *The China Study* — detailed in Chapter Four — showing that when carcinogens are present in the body, the rate of cancerous growth can be controlled by diet. They also discovered that liver cancer is more prevalent in those who diets were higher in animal protein (Campbell 2006). And, finally, they concluded that "only a tiny minority" of cancers can be solely blamed on one's genes.

Even Dr. Neal Barnard, President of the Physicians Committee for Responsible Medicine, says (Barnard 2001) that "if you change to a vegan diet . . . you can . . . prevent most cases of cancer."

Can You Believe It?

We Americans have been fed a myth, that we need animal protein to be healthy. Close Bible examination shows that after Adam and Eve sinned, the only items Yahweh added to man's diet were herbs and green vegetables. And it was after the flood, when man was given permission to eat flesh foods because the deluge had wiped out all vegetation, that man's life-span gradually grew shorter.

Copying the Ostrich

Also after the flood, Yahweh warned Noah that He would *require* the life of everyone who killed beasts or other men without cause. And if they had to eat flesh, because there was no abundant garden produce, they were to drain off the blood before preparing the flesh for food (Genesis 9:1-4).

Those people in a hurry to bury the Old Testament completely overlook the three NEW TESTAMENT admonitions about draining off the blood before preparing flesh food for consumption (Acts 15:20 + 29 and 21:25). This would eliminate beefsteak, most roasts, and hamburger from the Christian consumer's diet, wouldn't it?

Whom Do You Trust?

Through the years I've discovered that most of us believe what we *want* to, or what is *comfortable*, or what we *hope* is true. That reminds me of a project Dr. Veith, the zoology professor mentioned earlier, assigned his students. He told them that he believed carnivores could thrive on a vegetarian diet, and they laughed him to scorn.

However, when the results were in, they had to admit that not only did the flesh-eating animals do exceptionally well on their vegetarian fare, but their intestines also expanded so they could retain their food for a longer period, to absorb more nutrients from the plants they ate, the way human intestines do.

These results showed that, before the entrance of sin, ALL animals could have subsisted on grasses and greenery just as the Scripture says.

A Bloody Lie

When the World Cancer Research Fund, after a review of more than 7,000 clinical studies, issued a report saying processed meats – such as bacon, ham, salami, corned beef, and some sausages – were linked to a high risk of bowel cancer, the meat industry went ballistic, claiming the report was a "tool of the anti-meat lobby" (Physicians 2007).

Now consider this: Who stands to lose more money if consumers believe the report? The Research Fund, which is NOT in the meat and poultry business? Or the meat and dairy associations that can make a profit only if they convince people their products are essential for good health?

X-Rays and CAT Scans

There's much evidence to show that CAT scans, (often referred to as CT scans in the medical literature) are not always in our best interest. A couple years ago, the *Archives of Internal Medicine* estimated that 15,000 excess deaths from cancer were directly related to the increase in the number of CAT scans performed that year. This report was published after the "National Cancer Institute, Johns Hopkins University School of Medicine, and other medical centers conducted a study in 2007" (Secret 2011) and concluded that "CT scans performed in the US resulted in 29,000 new cancer cases a year."

Health Nuggets

But if you're already scheduled for a CAT scan with no other alternative for diagnosing a hidden ailment, note this: *The British Journal of Radiology* suggests taking "vitamins E, C, and beta-carotene" before undergoing ionizing radiation, to protect your cells from DNA damage caused by the procedure. These vitamins and minerals are prevalent in raw fruits and vegetables.

By the way, researchers were able to double the life span of laboratory mice which had begun to grow tumors by feeding them blueberry extract. Some of their tumors even shrank while the other mice, who weren't fed the extract, died (Hope-2 2011). If I had my choice, I'd choose blueberry extract over a CAT scan any day.

Also, if you're worried about cancer, a ten-year study on over 20,000 women (the well-known nurses' study) showed that those who ate more veggies, getting more fiber into their diets, reduced their risk of getting breast cancer by 15 percent (Hope-2 2011).

In addition, *The China Study* (Campbell 2006) found "the diet that prevents cancer is the same one that prevents heart disease, obesity, diabetes, cataracts, macular degeneration, Alzheimer's, cognitive dysfunction, multiple sclerosis, and osteoporosis."

Did that list include "diabetes"? Hmmm. Let's look at *that* research.

6. The King's Disease

*If thou wilt diligently hearken to the voice of the Lord
thy God, and wilt do that which is right in his sight,
and wilt give ear to his commandments, and keep all
his statutes, I will put none of these diseases upon thee,
which I have brought upon the Egyptians; for I am the
Lord that healeth thee.* — Exodus 15:26

While researching Egyptian customs before writing my
Biblical novel *Aaron's Rod,* I found that the ancient
Egyptians suffered the same diseases that plague Americans
today: heart disease, arthritis, gout, and diabetes.

Portly Royalty

Diabetes and gout often afflict people with big tummies
who eat a rich diet and sit around a lot. In Egypt diabetes was
called the "king's disease" because ants always congregated
around places where members of the royal family had urinated.
Being wealthier than the common people, royalty ate a much
richer diet. Records show that they even knew how to make ice
cream with snow imported from the mountains, and the ants were

drawn to the sugar in their urine! That could be why, for years, we thought people got diabetes from eating too much sugar.

Now we know differently. It's not sugar, but fat — present in our diets and found stored in our bodies — that causes the problem. This fat blocks the doorway to each cell in our bodies. These cells need insulin to help them absorb glucose from the blood. When the pancreas releases insulin, the insulin hurries to those cells but can't get in because the doorways are blocked (by fat), so they can't break down the sugar and convert it into usable glucose.

This is Type II diabetes — which was once called "adult-onset" diabetes — not Type I (juvenile diabetes), a completely different disease from the one discussed here.

"Nearly 24 million Americans have been diagnosed with diabetes" (NH 2010), and it's estimated that another 10 to 20 million Americans are either pre-diabetic or are already diabetic but haven't yet been diagnosed because their symptoms haven't become severe enough for them to seek medical attention.

Silent Stealth Bomber

Because diabetes often creeps up on people gradually and they don't notice a sudden decline in their health, it's often difficult to convince people that they really have the disease. That's what happened to Rayella's father:

Rayella couldn't convince her father to watch his diet. He'd been diagnosed with diabetes; but because he didn't feel sick, he wouldn't acknowledge that anything was wrong. He refused to begin exercising or make any changes in his diet — until one day when he got up too fast, lost his balance, fell, and couldn't get up.

Now he's in the hospital with a broken hip and must take insulin. If only he'd taken the diagnosis seriously, cut down on portions of fatty foods, increased his intake of fresh fruits and veggies, and started taking a daily walk! He probably could have controlled his blood sugar naturally and been able to indulge in an occasional treat. Now, however, his blood sugar will be carefully monitored, and he'll be forced to take insulin, whether he likes it or not.

Even though diabetes can sneak up on people, it's nothing to ignore. Currently, diabetes is (1) the United States' fifth leading cause of death by disease, (2) "a leading cause of heart disease and stroke," and (3) responsible for such tragedies as "adult blindness, kidney failure and non-traumatic amputations" (Diabetes 2010).

Recently Fox News reported that the death rate for diabetic women with breast cancer is "50 percent higher than that of non-diabetic women with breast cancer" (Fox 2011). Since diabetes is a "lifestyle related" disease and is never caused by pollution, as cancer is claimed to be, we should consider ourselves forewarned.

Choosing Your Medicine

Health institutes are springing up all over America, where people can go as inpatients, to reverse their diabetes. However, the disease returns unless people stay on the new lifestyle learned at the sanitarium. The physicians who run these institutions have all come to the conclusion that "if there is diabetes, then there is heart disease," a bit of news that should make us *all* eager to avoid becoming diabetic (Brackett 2006).

You'd think that natural cures for lifestyle-related diseases would be taught in all the medical schools, wouldn't you? I understand that physicians usually take only one course in nutrition, at most, in medical school. And we know several women who dropped out of nursing school when they discovered they'd be expected to know more about drugs than about real remedies.

One of these young women, after dropping out, married an epileptic man she'd met at college. We heard them give a musical performance while they were dating.

Several years later, we met them and their two little girls at a nearby park. The wife told me they were strict vegetarians, growing much of their own food. After leaving college she bought a book on herbal medicine, studied on her own, and periodically gave her husband the herbs recommended for preventing seizures. Since then, she claims he hasn't had any more symptoms.

Frank and I noticed that women who go through nursing school often place more reliance on doctors and drugs than they do on natural remedies. Of course, administering medications is part of their curriculum, but it saddens me when they believe physicians are smarter than Yahweh.

Apparently some ancient Egyptian doctors knew their stuff, though. Here's an inscription found carved on a tomb there: "Man lives on one-fourth of what he eats. On the other three-fourths lives his doctor" (Iglesias 1998).

Since diabetes is a *lifestyle-related* disease, we can usually prevent it by following certain health rules. Many practitioners claim that if people followed Yahweh's original meal plan and got plenty of exercise, diabetes would practically disappear from the American scene.

Although diabetics often go to special clinics to learn a healthier way to live, Frank and I know several people who got rid of their diabetes without leaving home.

Take Gloria's miraculous experience, for instance:

Gloria's Story

We met Gloria, a diabetic in her thirties, before we began seriously studying the Biblical health principles. Her brother had joined a Bible-believing church, so she began reading the Bible to see what it was all about. After a couple months, she was impressed that taking laboratory-produced insulin (a foreign substance not part of the Genesis diet) was not a good Biblical principle. So without telling her doctor, she changed to a vegetarian diet and stopped taking her insulin. When she went for her next appointment, the doctor found her blood sugar to be normal. He pronounced her cured and told her to "keep on doing what she was doing." She couldn't wait to tell us about the miracle God had performed.

It takes faith to make such a drastic change, and Gloria gave Yahweh all the credit. Her healing happened almost overnight — although it might have been a few weeks before she actually went for her medical checkup. And her recovery didn't occur because she had studied about the benefits of vegetarianism and exercise, either. She simply acted on what she'd read in the Old Testament.

Jack's Struggle

Jack, on the other hand, didn't act on anything he'd read in the Bible. A chef for many years, he'd been hearing about reversing diabetes the natural way, but felt it would be too much work to try to cook two different meals — one for his customers and a different, healthier one for himself. Although he was a vegetarian, he'd gained a lot of weight through the years and was exhausted most of the time. His doctor finally told him that if he didn't do something about his weight he'd end up in a wheelchair, or even the hospital, since the insulin shots didn't seem to be helping him. Apparently the doctor's words struck fear in Jack's heart because he resigned from his chef's position and went on a low-fat, mostly raw, vegan diet.

Previously, Jack had eaten lots of fried foods and meat analogs (nicknamed *veggie-meat*), but he quit eating both. His main goal was to lose weight, but he began experiencing other benefits. The first thing he noticed was that his blood sugar was more controllable; he felt better and was able to cut back on his insulin. Then he had to buy some new clothes, and he liked the way they fit. The longer he stuck to the program, the better he looked and felt.

His life changed so drastically, Jack became a new person at age 65! A lifelong bachelor, he has become more out-going and now has a girlfriend. He also discovered he likes to hike and be physically active, too.

We couldn't believe he was the same person when we bumped into Jack recently. He's so thrilled with his new look and energy that he's trying to convince his young diabetic friend Jeff to follow the program, too. So far, though, Jeff has resisted the offer. He believes Jack's regime is *too harsh*. Personally, I'd rather follow a healthful lifestyle — even if it requires learning new habits — than end up having to give myself insulin shots!

Jack's was not an overnight miracle, like Gloria's, but his diabetes has now reversed itself. He checks his blood sugar only occasionally, just to make sure he's not regressing.

According to the first Adventist Health Study, an intensive ten-year study of dietary habits of thousands of Californians in the 1970s, "those who consumed meat six or more days a week had a 3.8 times greater risk than vegetarians of dying of diabetes" (Snowden et al 1984).

This was corroborated in the July 2010 issue of the *Journal of Public Health Nutrition,* which reported that a study of over 75,000 Hawaiian adults aged 45 to 75, showed that "intake of red meat was positively associated with diabetes risk in men and women . . . and supports the growing evidence that red and processed meat intake increase risk for diabetes" (Cohen 2010).

But vegetarians can develop diabetes, too. We know several vegetarian diabetics who are overweight, follow no regular exercise program, and walk haltingly, as if their legs bother them.

Vicious Cycle

Studies show that diabetic medication gradually becomes ineffective if people don't control their food choices, and their doctors must keep prescribing a different medication. In addition, those medications only manage the symptoms; they don't cure the disease. Most well-informed doctors say diabetes medication, without a change in lifestyle, merely postpones the day that the patient has to begin taking insulin shots.

In 2003 a top executive of Glaxo-SmithKline pharmaceuticals admitted that "the vast majority of drugs — more than 90 percent — work only in 30 to 50 percent of the people." In fact, the same source (Easy 2011) reports that "the odds of being killed by conventional medicine [in the U.S.] are almost 20 times greater than being killed in an automobile accident."

So why do many physicians, who know about the natural way to reverse diabetes, still prescribe medicine for their patients when they know the drug only helps manage the symptoms? It's not because they don't care! After doctors have harped at a patient about losing weight for several months and they realize the patient isn't doing anything about it, they know very well the person isn't willing to change lifestyles and begin an exercise program. So they inwardly shake their heads in despair and write out a prescription, warning the patient that it's a downhill battle because most diabetes medications lose their effectiveness while the patient keeps abusing his body.

That's what happened to another friend of Frank's who wouldn't even listen to talk about reversing his diabetes the natural way. Visiting this friend in a nursing home and watching his health deteriorate, Frank was in tears every time we left there. This friend had both legs amputated in the year-and-a-half before he died.

Bible Prescriptions That Reverse Diabetes?

Does Yahweh heal our diseases without our even asking? Gloria didn't *ask* to be healed. She just determined she wasn't going to do anything that displeased Yahweh, like putting a nonfood substance in her body. On the other hand, Jack was thinking only of losing weight. Neither one attended a health clinic or institute, but both followed Biblical precepts and both were healed, even without praying for healing.

Yahweh's Promise of Healing

Yahweh gives several commands about draining off the blood when killing animals for consumption. Most of the cuts of meat I see in the grocery stores still contain blood. But the New Testament *three times* admonishes us not to eat the flesh of any animal that has been slain without draining off the blood (Acts 15:20+29 and 21:25). How can people who buy red meat over the counter claim to be NEW TESTAMENT Christians?

Everyone who has ever worried about a blood transfusion knows that disease can be transmitted through the blood. If the blood is diseased, who wants it entering his or her body? And we don't have to listen to the evening news very long before we realize the nation's meat supply grows more diseased every year.

Some people pray for healing but never experience the miracle. In the Bible verse at the beginning of the chapter, Yahweh says *He* does the healing, but He also gives certain conditions. Those conditions include obeying His *statutes*, so let's review a few.

If you want to avoid diabetes, or even if you're already diabetic, you can help yourself by making simple lifestyle changes. Beginning today —

•   Eat Yahweh's prescribed diet, consisting of fruits, nuts, and grains, prepared without too much adulteration. Have at least one big salad daily. In third world countries where "fast food" hasn't yet made an appearance, or where the people are too poor to dine out, diabetes is rare. And so are cancers, heart problems, and high blood pressure.

•   Keep physically active. Proverbs 6:6 calls people who don't work *sluggards*. And in Luke 12:20 Jesus called the man who decided to stop work and go into retirement a *fool*.

•   When you purchase flesh food, choose only those cuts which meet all Yahweh's requirements: (1) found on His "safe to eat" list, (2) drained of blood, and (3) sold with the fat cut off.

Frank was discussing animal fat and cholesterol with a dental surgeon lately. The dentist, a marathon runner, told Frank something interesting about animal fat. He said that if you don't cut it off *before* cooking the meat, the fat actually gets absorbed into the flesh itself, resulting in a double dose of dietary cholesterol.

Not good!

Young and Younger

Although it was once strictly an adult-onset disease, young children are now being diagnosed with Type II Diabetes. And that's because many of our children are obese. Their diets are fat-laden and they no longer exercise outdoors after school hours, as we did when we were growing up. In fact, researchers are telling us that, for the first time in American history, our children will have a shorter lifespan than we.

Desserts like ice cream, doughnuts, cakes, pies, cookies, fried dough, and other pastries contain both fat and sugar. Such desserts don't build muscle, don't add fiber to the diet, and don't keep the blood vessels and capillaries flexible, so these delicacies are great contributors to diabetes.

Since obese children as young as eight years old are now succumbing to diabetes; some of the contributors may be the Four White Poisons — covered in the next chapter.

7. The Four White Poisons

Be not desirous of [the king's] dainties, for they are deceitful meat. — Proverbs 20:1-3

Nothing can nourish our bodies as well as the whole foods that Yahweh pronounced *good*, like the original diet given in the Book of Genesis. In the days of the patriarch Abraham and his contemporaries, people stone-ground their grains into meal and flourished on the bread or cakes they baked with it. But sometime later, the aristocracy decided breads and cakes made with bleached flour were more appetizing. Whole grains were eventually considered peasant fare.

Soon white bread became a status symbol, even though many of the nutrients are removed in the bleaching process. As soon as the common people could afford to, they switched to white bread for their tables and white flour for their baking as well.

But a diet consisting mainly of breads and desserts baked with white, bleached flour can lead to sluggish bowels, hemorrhoids, and unwanted weight gain.

The Four White Poisons

For years, savvy nutritionists have called white flour, white sugar, white rice, and table salt *the four white poisons*. That's because these four processed white foods are often overused and cause many health problems. Breads, cereals, and pastas made from whole grains deliver more nutrition and dietary fiber than those made from bleached, refined flour.

One of the reasons people first lose weight on the high-protein/low-carbohydrate diet is because they previously ate mostly fried potato, white rice, and breads or other baked goods made with white flour and sugar. Such foods, which contain hardly any fiber, tend to clog our systems and lead to obesity. But brown rice and other whole grains contain beneficial fiber, usable protein, and many of the B vitamins which are lacking in flesh foods.

Healthy Brains Need Vitamin B

White sugar should rightly be called a *condiment*, rather than a food, and is discussed more thoroughly in the next chapter. Foods freely sweetened with sugar are an indirect cause of dental caries and, eaten in abundance, can lead to Vitamin B deficiencies and their related diseases.

Cancer, Parkinson's disease, and Alzheimer's are only three of the many conditions thought to be exacerbated by a lack of the B vitamins. Oxford University researchers conducted a study on elderly people with mild cognitive impairment and concluded that certain B vitamins — "folic acid, vitamin B-6, and B-12" — reduce brain shrinkage, a symptom of dementia (CBC News 2010). The above findings are good reasons to switch to whole grains.

My Favorite Poison

White rice, which I loved as a child, has had many of the natural vitamins and nutrients removed just as white flour has. The producers replace these health-giving nutrients with inorganic, laboratory-produced vitamins. But many nutritionists agree that people who eat large quantities of white rice often suffer from constipation and its many side effects including diverticulitis, acne, polyps, diabetes, hemorrhoids, gout, and colon cancer as well as unwanted weight gain.

In my teenage years I was prone to constipation; but switching to brown rice and other whole grains in my mid-twenties eliminated that problem. Brown rice contains more fiber and more usable protein than white rice, so it helps rid the body of toxins and other wastes too. That's probably why I started having more energy after I made the switch.

The Salt of the Earth

Our bodies need some salt, but many people overdo it. Some people are so addicted that they salt their food before they even taste it! A diet high in refined table salt leads to high blood pressure and makes the body retain fluid, especially in the elderly.

In the old days, salt was the only ingredient in our salt shakers, and it often clumped together in damp weather. But modern salt, which flows well in any climate, contains additives including sugar. Switching to mineral salt or sea salt, which costs more than the regular kind, has helped Frank and me cut down on the excessive use of table salt while increasing the minerals in our diet.

When we consume fresh fruit, vegetables, raw nuts, and whole grains — eliminating the four white poisons from our daily fare, we'll feel more energetic and experience fewer weight problems. That is, if we stay away from soda pop, packaged snacks, and processed foods containing artificial sweeteners!

Weightier Matters

As mentioned earlier, one reason people lose weight quickly when they first go on the high-protein/low-carbohydrate diet is because they are no longer eating white rice, white bread, and pastries made with white flour and sugar. They also cut back on potatoes slathered with butter or sour-cream topping. A diet consisting mainly of flesh foods, however, increases cholesterol and contributes to plaque build-up in the arteries. A later chapter in this book records the link between animal protein and kidney damage and shows that a high animal protein diet really isn't the wisest way to lose unwanted weight.

In fact, the *American Journal of Clinical Nutrition* recently reported that their study of meat eaters in ten European countries, including the UK, proved that people could lose weight merely by eating smaller portions of meat and larger helpings of vegetables and salads at each meal.

The study leader, Dr. Anne-Claire Vergnaud, suggests "cutting down on the amount of meat we eat" to avoid weight gain. The researchers further claim, "A portion of meat should be about the size of a deck of cards" (BBC news 2010).

Deter Diabetes in Children

To deter diabetes in their families, parents should encourage their children to —

- Exercise daily. Limit their time in front of computers and television sets.
- Learn to enjoy brown rice and whole-grain breads.
- Choose a piece of fresh fruit, a handful of raisins, or carrot and celery sticks if snacking between meals.

In addition, avoid feeding children the four white poisons. Serve whole foods as they're grown, without refining them and removing all the nutrition. (Genesis 1:29)

Prepare vegetables in a variety of ways and serve less meat at the table: A handful of raw almonds, walnuts, or sunflower seeds will provide any meal's requirement for protein.

Limit your children's sugar intake. Too much can cause havoc as we'll see in the next chapter.

8. Sweets for the Sweet

Hast thou found honey? Eat so much as is sufficient for thee, lest thou be filled therewith, and vomit it. — Proverbs 25:16

It is not good to eat much honey.
— Proverbs 25:27

According to the above texts, we should be eating only enough honey to supply our needs. Whether it's in the comb or bottled, though, honey can be rather messy; so most Americans prefer to keep a sugar bowl handy.

Because we can buy refined sugar at the grocery store, we tend to use more than we should. Too much refined sugar can suppress the immune system, produce a significant rise in triglycerides, lead to chromium deficiency, increase the systolic blood pressure, cause cataracts, damage the pancreas, deepen depression, multiply the risk of getting gout, exacerbate PMS, worsen ADHD symptoms, advance gum disease, and induce cell death (Appleton 2004).

Another reason to limit sugary desserts is because Candida is becoming rampant in our society. According to the

Sugar Shock lady, sugar is the "number one contributor to Candida" (Bennett 2010), although wheat flour, baker's yeast, and milk products seem to worsen the problem.

Misguided Me

Whole books have been written about the dangers of using artificial sweeteners, so when I read that fructose was a "natural" sugar and could be used in cooking, I bought a batch of fructose powder and began cooking with that, believing I was using a health food. A while later, though, I learned that fructose is very healthful while it's still in its natural state in a piece of fruit. But when extracted from fruit, transformed into a refined sweetener, and used freely, it's even more damaging than plain table sugar.

Trying to make healthful desserts can be frustrating. And seeing the variety of sweeteners on the grocery shelves can cause much confusion. Here are a number of common refined sugars and their original sources.

- Sucrose, often also spelled succharose, is derived from sugar cane, sugar beets, or a combination of both.
- Dextrose, sometimes wrongly called glucose, is extracted from corn.
- Lactose is milk sugar, found in cow's milk. Apparently it can be manufactured from other

products as well, since some ingredient labels claim their lactose is from non-dairy sources.

- Maltose (a.k.a. "malt") is malt sugar, made from fermented barley used in brewing beer, OR from sprouted corn or wheat, so people sensitive to wheat should ask its source before buying products containing malt.

- Fructose is fruit sugar, naturally occurring in fruit. But if it's HFCS (high fructose corn syrup), it's been through a chemical process using genetically modified corn and may contain toxic levels of mercury.

- Glucose is blood sugar, supplying energy for the brain. It's produced in our bodies; obtained from the fruits, veggies, grains, and legumes we eat; and regulated by the pancreas. Any excess sugar the body can't use gets stored in fat cells.

After leaving the stomach, most sugars enter the blood stream as glucose, and the pancreas sends out insulin to regulate its use in our bodies. But HFCS is different. It doesn't get broken down until it reaches our liver. And since there's no insulin in our liver to handle it, the HFCS gets turned into triglycerides which have been implicated in heart attacks.

Ask my husband. He'll tell you! When Frank had his heart attack, his cholesterol readings were normal. The only problem the doctors could find was an abnormally high triglyceride count. That knowledge didn't ease his pain, though.

In March 2011, the Corn Refiners Association appealed to the FDA for permission to label HFCS as "corn sugar" because many people have stopped buying products containing HFCS. Be forewarned, though, that if in the future you read *corn sugar* on a label, it'll still be high fructose corn syrup. Also, when consumers complained about its being labeled *corn sugar*, rumor has it that the FDA has given them permission to call it *beet sugar*. Buyers beware!

The Old Plantation

Long ago dentists noticed that people who couldn't afford to buy table sugar had no dental caries. Only the wealthy plantation owners and their families, who had sugar bowls and who sweetened their cereals and fruit with refined sugar, suffered from dental problems. Yet the natives chewed on sugar cane while they worked in the fields, and their teeth and gums remained strong. So, for years, dentists claimed refined sugar caused cavities.

But that's only a half-truth. What refined sugar does is change our systems from alkaline-base to acid-base. If we eat large amounts of fresh fruits and veggies, our systems remain alkaline, and harmful bacteria cannot thrive in our mouths. But soda pop, candy bars, meat, and processed foods tip our systems toward the acid side. The bacteria which cause cavities thrive

ONLY in an acid environment. Brushing our teeth and scraping our tongues will leave our mouths feeling fresh and clean, but those activities can't change an acid system to an alkaline one. Only a diet containing alkaline-base foods can do that.

Yahweh said our bread and water would be sure, but he never told us to eat sugar-laden desserts. For special occasions, I sometimes make a simple dessert sweetened with dates, banana, or concentrated fruit juice. Generally, though, Frank and I avoid desserts in an effort to keep our systems alkaline.

As a teenager I drank too much soda pop; and by the time I was twenty-five, I had a mouth full of fillings. But after we simplified our diet, eating an abundance of fresh fruits and veggies and eliminating refined sugars, I stopped getting cavities.

Natural Sweeteners

Several natural sweeteners are now sold in health food stores: honey, maple syrup, stevia, agave, and XyloSweet®, to name a few. The latter three supposedly have a low glycemic index and can be safely used by diabetics. The Indians used stevia, harvested from an herb called "sweet leaf," as a sweetener. Xylitol® breath mints leave the mouth alkaline, so there's no danger of cavities.

But Xylitol® comes from corn cobs; and most corn grown in the U.S. is now genetically modified (Northstar 2011). If you're avoiding GMOs (genetically modified foods), you might want to question the source of any Xylitol® products you purchase (Northstar 2011).

Regarding agave, Dr. Mercola warns us that some syrups labeled *Agave* contain as much as 80 percent fructose. If we use the sweetener, we should know the process used in its extraction from the agave plant and its preparation for bottling because the following chemicals may be used in the syrup's production: "Activated charcoal, cationic and tonic resins, sulfuric and/or hydrofluoric acid, dicalite, clarimex, inulin enzymes, and fructozyme" (Mercola 2011).

Remember, though, that these newer sweeteners are all refined, just like white sugar, processed honey, and maple syrup; they're NOT whole foods.

Ohio allergist Dr. John Boyles considers genetically modified foods so dangerous he cautions his patients' families to stay away from them. An AAEM position paper blames GMO animal feed for "infertility, immune dysregulation . . . and changes in the liver, kidney, spleen and gastrointestinal system" (AD 2005). Amazing Discoveries® also reports what happened to some laboratory rats which were fed GMO soy: The male rats' testicles changed from their normal pink color to a dark blue. The female rats either aborted their fetuses or lost their babies right after delivery. Pig farmers have reported false pregnancies, sterility, and their pigs' "giving birth to bags of water" after eating a steady diet of GMO corn feed.

Seed developers like Monsanto® and other producers of GMO foods pooh-pooh the idea that GMOs could be harmful. But many a scientist has become "a voice crying in the wilderness" against them. As for me, I ponder who will make the most $$ profit from those products and tend to side with the lone scientist who's studied enough of the research to be scared for his family's health.

Side Effects

All drugs made in a laboratory have side effects, and artificial sweeteners are no exception. While attending a night class many years ago, I got sick after eating a small bag of sugarless candies sweetened with an artificial sweetener, and it was no picnic!

In our house, I keep a little brown sugar in my sugar bowl, mostly as a conversational piece. If I'm serving an herbal tea to guests who depend on artificial sweeteners, it gives me a chance to explain the dangers of sugar substitutes and urge them to switch to a more healthful sweetener while cutting down on their sugar intake.

Some people use Splenda® regularly. But studies report its side effects to include diarrhea, shrunken thymus glands, enlarged liver and kidneys, decreased red blood cell count, hyperplasia of the pelvis, extension of the pregnancy period, aborted pregnancy, and decreased fetal body and placental weights (Hull 2010).

Aspartame®, which frequently goes under some other names including AminoSweet®, NutraSweet®, and Equal®, is *not* a healthful sweetener. When exposed to heat for long periods (like sitting outdoors on a hot day), some of the chemical components in Aspartame® turn into formaldehyde, the

substance used in embalming fluid. Side effects of Aspartame®
can include "headache, change in vision, convulsions and
seizures, hallucination, nausea and vomiting, and joint pain"
(Mercola 2010).

For a more complete run-down on the side effects of
artificial sweeteners, visit Dr. Mercola's web site listed in the
bibliography.

Some soft drink manufacturers claim they are switching
to stevia, to make their beverages healthier. But be careful.
They're not using the whole herb as the native Indians did.
They're actually using erythritol, an extract of stevia, which is
mixed with crystalline fructose and sucrose. So although it
sounds like an herbal sweetener, this additive is just another
artificial sweetener. It's no longer in its natural state, and it's
NOT a whole food.

The two major American soda pop manufacturers plan to
use a zero-calorie sweetener called *rebiana*, another synthetic
mixture containing an extract from the stevia plant, to replace
Aspartame® in their diet drinks. That is, until the public
complains. When sales drop, these producers will change the
names again, as they've previously done with Aspartame®, to
fool consumers into thinking their drinks are good for people.

The safest course is to give up all foods containing
artificial sweeteners. Most people who drink the diet sodas for
any length of time find they can't maintain a steady weight.

Studies have shown that artificial sweeteners actually stimulate our appetites and make us eat and drink more.

A recent report from the American Diabetes Association claims that people who drank diet soda over a ten-year period had waist circumference increases 500 percent greater than people who didn't drink the stuff. And some folks claim they've lost up to seventeen pounds, without going on a diet, simply by giving up diet drinks and switching to plain water between meals.

In addition, one health organization also reported that longtime ingestion of diet sodas usually leads to Type II Diabetes.

What's the Harm?

Regular soda pop may be less harmful than diet sodas. But not much. Some researchers found that not only is refined sugar a "culprit in diabetes, heart disease, and strokes" (Spector 2010), but it also appears to have a direct correlation to cancer of the pancreas, one of the deadliest cancers there is.

A report in *Cancer Epidemiology, Biomarkers & Prevention* on a 14-year study in Singapore, involving over 60,000 subjects, showed that those "who drank two or more soft drinks a week had an 87 percent higher risk" of getting pancreatic cancer (O'Callahan 2010).

The five-year survival rate for pancreatic cancer is about five percent. And while some studies have linked this cancer to red meat, especially burned or charred, the *Journal of Cancer Research* found that pancreatic "cancer cells feed easily on . . .

fructose, and that the sugar helps the cells proliferate" (Spector 2010).

In the United States, over 37,000 people are diagnosed with pancreatic cancer each year, and over 34,000 die from it. In February 2010, yahoo readers were warned that tests showed tumor cells thrive on sugar. In fact, "tumor cells use more glucose than other cells." And a twelve-ounce can of regular soda contains "about 130 calories, almost all of them from sugar" (Jonsson 2010).

Switching to diet sodas is not the answer, though. Remember that some of the artificial sweeteners contain high fructose corn syrup. Researchers at UCLA's Jonsson Cancer Center compared fructose with glucose and discovered that cancer cells love fructose even MORE than they do glucose.

In addition, a recent study found that drinking sweetened drinks such as fruit juices, iced tea, and sports beverages can increase a person's risk of developing diabetes by 26 percent. "Sugar-loaded drinks deliver a quick rush of sugars to your body, which over time can lead to insulin resistance and inflammation, explains Jacob Teitelbaum, MD, author of *Beat Sugar Addiction"* (fitbie 2011).

Help Yourself to Better Health

Many people wash their food down with some type of liquid at mealtimes. These simple changes in habit will bring manifold blessings:

1. Chew your food thoroughly and avoid washing it down with any liquid. (Prevents overeating.)
2. If you must drink with your meal, choose only water. (Automatically cuts calories.)
3. Drink plenty of water between meals. (Cuts down hunger pangs.)
4. At parties and receptions, drink the punch first, and give it a few minutes to digest before tackling the solid foods. (Activates people's *appestat* and prevents overeating.)

We would do our kidneys, liver, and pancreas a favor if we gave up soft drinks entirely and drank just water. Water is....

- natural — sometimes,
- free — in many cases, and
- a pain fighter — as we'll see in the next chapter.

9. The Water of Life

*In the last day, that great day of the feast, Jesus
stood and cried, saying, "If any man thirst, let
him come unto me, and drink. He that believeth
on me, as the scripture hath said, out of his belly
shall flow rivers of living water."*
— John 7:37-38

Why did Christ say he was the "water of life"? Why not the
wine or grape juice of life? Could it be because not only
is water the best thirst quencher on the planet, but also because
every cell in our body needs a daily water bath for optimal
function?

Yahweh tells us that, when times are bad, our bread and
water will be sure. According to the Bible, bread and water are
basic necessities of life. I've met a few people, though, who drink
water only when there's no other beverage available. And yet –

Medical Miracle

While serving as a political inmate during the Iranian
Revolution in 1979, Dr. Batman (short for Batmanghelidj) was
put in charge of the medical dispensary there. One day an ulcer

patient in extreme pain came to his dispensary for help, but they'd run out of medicine for peptic ulcers. Stalling for time, while he tried to think of an alternative medication, Dr. Batman gave the patient two glasses of water. And then, because no solution came to his mind, he gave him another. A few minutes later, he realized the patient had stopped moaning and was no longer bent over in pain. To his surprise, as well as the patient's, the pain was gone.

After that, Dr. Batman repeated the water treatment whenever an ulcer patient came to his dispensary in pain. And the same miracle occurred every time! In fact, as long as the patients kept drinking plenty of water, their ulcers didn't return. When Batman left the prison, he began experimenting with other ailments and discovered many of them also cleared up when the patients began drinking water regularly. After years of study on water's curative qualities, he concluded that many diseases are caused by chronic dehydration.

His first book *Your Body's Many Cries for Water* was published in 1992, and he later wrote *UCD: A New Medical Discovery,* which he hoped would change the way the medical establishment treated disease. He believed chronic dehydration is the cause of much "pain and disease, including cancer in the body." However, there's no money to be made by physicians and drug companies with such a simple, inexpensive cure as water. So, even though many copies of his book have sold, Batman's vision for a change in America's medical system will probably never come true this side of heaven.

I Saw the Light

Growing up, I read in my health class that we should drink eight glasses of water a day. But I discovered that drinking water sent me to the restroom often, so I decided the "eight-glasses-a-day" rule was okay for everyone else, but not for me. And I paid the price! By the time I was twenty-eight, I'd already suffered from two bladder infections and ended up with a weak kidney. A naturopathic doctor scolded me and suggested I get my act together.

So *now* I set my timer to remind me to drink water when I'm involved in a project. And I keep the day's supply in a see-through pitcher so I can pace myself and know when I've had my 50 ounces. We can't always teach an old dog new tricks, but having a weak kidney has convinced me that Yahweh's health principles were meant for ME as well as for the rest of His children.

Although some doctors claim that we lose our sense of thirst as we grow older, Dr. Kim firmly believes that "most people who are chronically dehydrated have learned to ignore a parched mouth" (Dr. Kim 2011). And that was certainly the predicament I found myself in when the naturopath set me straight.

Symptoms of Dehydration

Until reading Dr. Batman's first book (Batman 1992), I didn't realize the impact drinking water could have on my health. When I was going through my "water-makes-you-use-the-bathroom-more-often" stage, I often suffered dizziness when I'd have to stand still on a table so the dressmaker could pin the hems of my dancing costumes. But after I began drinking water regularly, I realized my dizzy spells had become a thing of the past.

According to Batman, abnormal fear of heights is also a sign of dehydration, and my father is a prime example. He started drinking coffee in his teenage years, but hardly ever drank water. When he drove with a group of friends to the top of a mountain to look at the view, my father wouldn't stand near the edge with the others. He stayed back five or six feet where he insisted he could see just fine. And he wouldn't climb fire towers, either, which we often do when we want a better view of the scenery.

My parents gave up coffee drinking when they learned caffeine was harmful to the body. But instead of drinking water, Dad switched to milk. And to his dying day, he avoided heights. He never even climbed ladders, but always hired a relative to come and change our storm windows or make home repairs above shoulder level.

In addition to fearing heights, my father had ulcers several times in his life. If only Dr. Batman had written his book

96

earlier, Dad might have gotten rid of his pain and — if he'd begun drinking water — prevented the recurrences.

Dr. Batman also claimed that *many* phobias were actually caused by dehydration; and the worse the dehydration, the more extreme would be the phobia. Peggy's agoraphobia certainly fits his description; he could have used her for one of his case histories, too. Peggy didn't like the taste of water and never drank it plain. She drank either coffee or milk with her meals and, following a heart attack in her late sixties, she developed agoraphobia (fear of going out in public).

At first, Tom was able to convince her to go on a Sunday drive with him if one of us neighbors promised to keep an eye on the house. But as time passed, she became more fearful and wouldn't leave the house at all, even with Tom. Though they both loved the smell of line-dried laundry, he had to buy an electric dryer because she wouldn't even step onto the porch to hang a dish towel. Before she went to the hospital for the last time, he had to ask a neighbor to sit with her while he went shopping or ran errands.

Tom wasn't the kind of person to complain to a doctor about his wife's strange behavior, and she refused to go for any medical visits, so she was never *officially* diagnosed as agoraphobia. Her cause of death was listed as kidney failure, but it doesn't take a rocket science to recognize the symptoms. Dr. Batman would have put her on a water-drinking regime (Batman 1992).

About the same time Peggy was dying, another friend of ours suffered with kidney problems.

"Can't your physician give you something for the pain," I asked.

"The medicine didn't agree with me," she said. "So he's giving me some herbal remedies. But he said it took years to get this way, and it won't go away overnight."

Unfortunately, this friend was killed in a car accident before I read Dr. Batman's book, so I couldn't share his water cures with her. I don't remember ever seeing her drink a glass of water, but it might have eased her pain while her kidneys were healing. I, for one, have REALLY benefited from drinking water.

Quick Fix for Back Strain

According to some authorities, even a two-percent drop in body water can trigger "fuzzy short-term memory, trouble with basic math, and difficulty focusing on the computer screen or on a printed page."

I haven't had any trouble with fuzzy thinking, but I've often used Dr. Batman's remedy after raking leaves or pruning bushes. Whenever I come indoors with a backache, brought on by heavy yard-work, I can usually ease the pain by drinking three glasses of water, about 15 minutes apart.

Other researchers besides Dr. Batman have suggested that 8 to 10 glasses of water a day could significantly ease back discomfort and lessen joint pain for up to 80 percent of sufferers.

Morning Shower or Evening Bath?

Several years ago I was telling a nutritionist that Sheila, one of my acquaintances, doesn't like the taste of water. And her doctor told her it was okay to drink orange juice instead.

The health practitioner snorted and asked, "Would you take a bath in orange juice? That's what you're doing to the cells in your body when you drink any other liquid besides water!"

Sheila has arthritis in her legs and back. In the three years they lived near us, she fell twice — once breaking her elbow and once cracking her shoulder bone. She and her husband have since relocated, but the last time I saw her she still believed orange juice with breakfast, soda pop with lunch, and a glass of milk with dinner supplied all her body's daily requirement for water.

Most medical doctors study only a smattering of nutrition in medical school. Their main focus is usually on diagnosing and treating illness, not preventing disease. Often, too, their advice contradicts that of researchers and experts in the field of nutrition. At least the Bible, if we let it interpret itself, is consistent.

Kidney Punch

Although Dr. Batman attributed many kidney problems to early stages of dehydration, the American Academy of Family Physicians notes that "high animal-protein intake is largely responsible for the high prevalence of kidney stones in the United states . . . and recommends protein restriction for the prevention of recurrent kidney stones" (Goldfarb 1999).

Many doctors are reporting kidney problems in patients who've stayed a long time on a *high-protein/low-carbohydrate* weight-loss program. One medical office reported ten percent of such dieters suffering from kidney stones, one percent having severe kidney infections, and eight percent operating with reduced kidney function.

One patient reported "recurring kidney infections with elevated leukocytes and blood in my urine" accompanied by much pain. Another had "three kidney stone episodes in the four months" that he was on the high animal-protein diet.

Still another patient experienced her first kidney stone episode while on a high animal-protein diet. "Even though I lost weight on the diet, if it's responsible for my . . . kidney stones, it's not worth it!" she declared (Your Health 2011).

A high animal-protein diet causes "excess protein molecules to be sent into the blood and through the kidneys, forcing them to work harder. The opposite has been true of people who eat a high plant-protein diet. Therefore, people with kidney problems should NOT eat high [animal] protein diets" (AARP 2011).

Which Stage?

Another study, unrelated to the previously mentioned one, found that excess proteins caused damage only in those people who already had mild kidney problems (Knight et al 2003). But a 2003 survey showed that more than 40 percent of Americans over age forty have reduced kidney function and don't even know it (Coresh et al 2003).

Kidney disease falls into five stages, and the first two don't usually exhibit any noticeable symptoms. Unless we go to the doctor's office for some other problem and have a blood test, we may not know our kidneys aren't operating at peak performance. That was MY experience. It was during a routine visit to a naturopath that my weak kidney was diagnosed. And that was a complete surprise, since I hadn't noticed any difference in my energy level.

Even in Stage Three kidney dysfunction, known as *moderate chronic renal insufficiency*, we may not experience any symptoms, although many folks are anemic, tire easily, and have some swelling from fluids by the time they reach this stage (Livestrong 2011).

Our vegetarian friend Roy suffered from occasional kidney stones. So of course we couldn't blame the protein from flesh foods for his stones, could we? Was he a little dehydrated, which put extra pressure on his kidneys? Or did he go overboard on synthetic meat substitutes? Probably both, since he wouldn't drink water and he loved his veggie-meat — which contains many acid-forming additives. Just read the labels and see for yourself.

If excess animal protein places a burden on our kidneys, imagine the added strain we put on them when we eat the flesh of *diseased* and *chemically-fed* animals!

Speaking of chemically-fed animals, two Central Minnesota dairy farmers were sent warning letters from federal officials in 2009 because their cows contained "129 times the amount of penicillin [neomycin] allowed" (Cohen 2009). "Neomycin is an antibiotic used to treat mastitis in cows. And although it's sometimes given orally, neomycin is never administered to humans intravenously because it causes kidney damage." It also overloads milk drinkers' systems with antibiotics. It's no wonder, then, that people who use a lot of dairy products often suffer from infections that are antibiotic-resistant (Cohen 2009). Some people substitute soda pop, coffee, and tea for water. After all, they're liquids, aren't they?

All Dried Up!

Soda pop, coffee, tea, and beer don't replace our body's requirements for water because they are "major dehydrating agents" (Journal H 2009). All caffeinated drinks pull water out of our cells to help flush the drug (caffeine or alcohol) from our kidneys.

Since our brains are 70 percent water, guess which cells get robbed first when we don't keep well hydrated? Of course, it's our brains! It's no wonder fuzzy thinking and difficulty making decisions are signs of mild dehydration.

In addition, soda pop has been blamed for the following problems:

- OBESITY - A Harvard medical study found that twelve-year-old boys who regularly drank soft drinks were "more likely to be overweight than those who didn't."
- TOOTH DECAY - Besides tipping our systems from alkaline to acid and creating an environment for bacteria to grow on the teeth, the acids in soda pop begin dissolving tooth enamel in "only twenty minutes" according to the Ohio Dental Association.
- CAFFEINE DEPENDENCE - Many soda pop formulas contain tiny amounts of caffeine, to assure a stronger taste and an energy rush.
- WEAKENED BONES - A 1994 Harvard study of bone fractures in teenage athletes found a strong association between cola beverage consumption and bone fractures. Fourteen-year-old girls who drank cola were about "five times more likely to suffer bone fractures than girls who didn't consume soda pop" (Squires 2001).

Yet, according to a 2001 *Washington Post* article, fifty-six percent of eight-year-olds "down soft drinks daily, and a third of teenage boys drink at least three cans of soda pop per day."

Another writer claims the average American drinks more than 60 gallons of soft drinks each year. Oops! Since I don't touch the stuff, this means the person drinking BOTH my share AND hers gets 120 gallons! Have you ever measured how much soda pop you drink?

Check off your soda pop intake below:

1) Only on the weekends (3-4 cans) _____

2) About three 12-oz. cans a week _____

3) One 12-oz. can each day _____

4) Two cans a day, with meals _____

5) More than two cans a day _____

Dr. Mercola has been warning people about the dangers of soda pop for over twelve years now. He considers it "one of the worst drinks a person can consume" (2011). Compare the items you checked with the following results Mercola has found from various studies:

(1 & 2) The high phosphoric acid content in a single can of soda pop causes changes in a person's urine. Mercola reports that a quart of soda per week "may increase your risk of developing kidney stones by 15 percent" (2011).

(3) Are you overweight? Drinking only one can a day "translates to more than a pound of weight gain every month!"

Some people believe that because soda pop makes us burp, it's actually settling our stomach. But that isn't really true. Soda pop often causes heartburn and can lead to acid reflux problems. In addition, the phosphoric acid in soda pop disturbs the acid-alkaline balance of the stomach and may lead to cancers in the digestive system.

(4) Do you drink two cans a day? Regular soda pop, twice a day, raises one's risk of developing gout by 85 percent. If the drinks are artificially sweetened with fructose, drinking two cans a day can cause stomach inflammation, contribute to weight gain, and trigger diabetes (Mercola 2011).

(5) According to Dr. Mercola, continual intake of cola-type drinks can also lead to caffeine intoxication, which is rarely discussed. A few of the symptoms are nervousness, insomnia, stomach upsets, tremors, rapid heartbeats, and restlessness. But he says that even drinking caffeine-free sodas on a regular basis can lead to a potassium deficiency.

No Need to Apologize

Last year I was apologizing to our family dentist for all the saliva that collects in my mouth when he's working on my teeth.

He laughed and said, "Actually, having a lot of saliva is a sign of good health. Dry mouth is a sign of cancer."

I should have asked him if he'd read Dr. Batman's books. Batman wrote, "Stress, headache, back pain, allergies, asthma, high blood pressure, and many degenerative health problems are the result of UCD, Unintentional Chronic Dehydration." He also claimed that dry mouth is a sign of *extreme* dehydration (Batman 2004).

According to Batman, even slight dehydration causes "decreased coordination, fatigue, dry skin, decreased urine output, dry mucus membranes in the mouth and nose, blood pressure changes, and impaired judgment."

The cells in our bodies are not like piggy banks that can be emptied completely, ignored for several months, and then refilled when the mood hits us. "When dehydration has become symptom-producing, the reversal of its complications takes time and understanding" (Batman 2004).

Timely Tip

Years ago I came across a great remedy for sluggish bowels, and I highly recommend it. Just drink two glasses of warm water on an empty stomach, first thing in the morning. It should move things right along and set the tone for the rest of your day.

If you get busy and forget to drink during the day, you might make a habit of following this daily program, suggested by a nutritionist: "Take two glasses of water upon arising, to activate the internal organs. Then drink a glass of water thirty minutes before each meal, to help digestion. If taking a bath, drink a glass of water beforehand, to help lower your blood pressure; and drink a glass of water before going to bed, to prevent stroke and a heart attack."

This habit will assure you at least five or six glasses of water a day, the absolute minimum, according to many health practitioners.

Just five glasses of water a day —
— Decreases the risk of colon cancer by 45%
— Can slash the risk of breast cancer by 79%
— Cuts the risk of developing bladder cancer by 50%

Heart-attack survivors can also reduce the risk of a fatal stroke by drinking water every day.

Liver Aide

For those who don't like plain water, a squirt of lemon or lime juice can give it a more pleasing taste. Restaurants serve water goblets decorated with a lemon or lime slice not only to make it look more elegant, but also to add a fresh flavor to an ordinary-tasting beverage. A tablespoon of lemon juice in a glass of warm water is a good liver tonic, too, especially if taken on an empty stomach first thing in the morning.

Inexpensive Water Cure

I haven't had a head-cold in ages, but in the days when I often did, a friend suggested a natural cure using only water. This remedy must be started as soon as you realize you're coming down with a cold: Set your timer and drink an eight-oz. glass of water every half hour.

This treatment might make you a little drowsy, so if you can lie down, a little nap between drinks doesn't hurt. It has always worked for me.

In fact, one day while working for a temporary agency years ago, I felt I must go in to the office even though I was coming down with a cold. The other lady in the office laughed when she saw me drinking so much water (and it didn't send me to the restroom every few minutes, either. I must have been dehydrated and didn't know it).

Anyway, I slept well that night and was back at the office the next day feeling fine. As stated earlier, this remedy works best at the first sign of a cold, not after the person's been sick a few days.

Let's leave our kidneys now, and look at a different part of our wonderfully made bodies!

10. The Three "F" Formula

Thou shalt not seethe a kid in his mother's milk.
— Ex. 23:19 & 34:26; Deut. 14:21

Some theologians insist this verse is merely an injunction against a pagan worship ritual that involved killing a baby goat and cooking it in its mother's milk. And since God's people are warned not to follow any of the pagan customs, they're at least partly correct.

The PETA people (People for the Ethical Treatment of Animals) claim the text is not just a prohibition against adopting pagan customs, but also an animal rights issue. They protest, "How inhumane it is to kill an animal and then add injury to the mother's anguish by cooking it in her own milk!"

And both these schools of thought have merit. But Yahweh, being smarter than we are, is able to teach more than one concept at a time. Besides being a moral teaching against copying pagan rituals and a mental directive fostering humane attitudes toward animals, this text also reinforces a physical wellness principle: Meat served with milk gravy is a dietary practice which has long been linked to gallbladder disease.

What Gall!

Back in the fifties, physicians had a cliché for diagnosing gallbladder disease. If a patient with stomach problems was "fair (skinned), fat, and forty," one of the first questions to ask would be, "Do you eat much gravy?"

If the answer was "yes," the doctors could be fairly sure they were dealing with a gallbladder issue.

In the 1970s, this *Three F Formula* got revamped from three Fs to five Fs: Then it was a "<u>F</u>at, <u>F</u>air, <u>F</u>latulent, <u>F</u>emale of <u>F</u>orty" who eats a rich diet and doesn't exercise regularly.

Today, though, doctors are omitting two of the <u>F</u>s: the one for <u>forty</u> is no longer a valid factor because people in their mid-twenties also experience gallbladder problems (Van Staten 2010). The <u>F</u> for <u>F</u>emale is also being discarded because an increasing number of males are being afflicted these days.

The *righthealth* web site claims the disease "commonly affects overweight people as a result of high blood cholesterol levels." A group of researchers found that gallbladder disease is absent in some groups of peoples in Asia and Africa. Blaming the more prevalent groups of gall bladder sufferers on "genetic" factors, the researchers didn't look into the diets of those groups where the disease and gallbladder stones are rare (Best P 2006). If they had, they might have discovered that those tribes in Asia and Africa don't pour milk-gravy over their meat before eating it.

Many researchers claim that eating foods rich in fat contribute to the disease's development (AARP and R. G. Stone). When we eat mashed potatoes with meat and gravy, whether it's goat meat or any other kind of flesh food, we're getting plenty of saturated animal fat and dietary cholesterol in our meal.

Who Knew?

Years ago when I was operating my dancing school up North, Cindy's father brought her to her tap-dancing lesson one day.

"Where's your wife?" I asked him, since it was usually she who brought Cindy to her lessons.

"She's in the hospital with our new baby."

"What?" I was shocked! Emma hadn't told anyone she was expecting. She was a very large woman, and we thought she was just overweight.

"Yes, we were all surprised. Even the doctor," her husband said.

As I mentioned, Emma was very heavy, and she didn't look much thinner when she resumed bringing Cindy to her lessons, either.

A few months later Cindy's father brought her to class again. This time Emma was in the hospital having her gallbladder removed.

Sometime later, I stopped in at their house on an errand, and I saw what Emma was preparing for supper – mashed potatoes, pot roast, and meat gravy. She definitely fit the *Five-F Formula*!

Of course, there are exceptions to every rule, but I've only met a couple slim people who've had gallbladder trouble. The two I knew were very picky eaters, usually pushing their vegetables aside and eating only the meat. To their credit, they chose small portions of dessert. As I said, they were fairly slim.

But those were exceptions. As a rule, most gallbladder victims are not slim and trim.

So Much Sauce

According to Van Straten (2010), an osteopath who's treated many classical musicians and popular athletes in the U.K., "The best way to prevent gallstones is to be a vegetarian." He claims they're "only half as likely to suffer [from gallbladder problems] as meat-eaters."

That may be true, but vegetarians can develop painful gallstones, too. And, as my husband can testify, women are NOT the only ones who suffer with them. Frank was a vegetarian when he was struck down, and he loved mashed potatoes with gravy, as well as other foods cooked in rich sauces. He also loved casseroles, especially those swathed in cheese sauce, and he indulged in them as often as he could.

Gallbladder disease is more common in European and American countries, where the diet is richer than in third-world countries. While some researchers blame genetic factors as well as environmental ones, the disease has a low prevalence in Asia and Africa, as mentioned earlier. Gastroenterologists noted that these people eat plenty of whole-grain carbohydrates with lots of fiber but not much fat, while the American and European diet contains more fat and processed carbohydrates but very little fiber. And the average Westerner tends to get less exercise, too (Best P 2006).

Van Straten warns that, besides a possible connection between gallbladder disease and taking oral contraceptives, "alternating between drastic diets and bingeing, with quick fluctuations in weight" can also be a contributing factor in gallbladder disease (2010).

The research shows that if we followed Yahweh's original diet and obeyed his statutes, we wouldn't suffer from many lifestyle-related physical ailments. And that includes gallbladder disease.

Liar, Liar, Pants on Fire!

It's been said that if you tell a whopper of a lie long enough and loud enough, after a while people will start to believe it. That's what happened after the original apostles died, when church leaders told the people in the pews that *torah* meant "law," rather than "teachings." Imagine the number of people who've died during gallbladder attacks through the centuries, not realizing that Yahweh's teachings are health to our bodies as well as to our souls!

On a secular scale the same scenario is happening in America's food and health-care industries, with skewed studies sponsored by special interest groups who make their living from the meat, dairy, and pharmaceutical industries. Some greedy manufacturers will pay a hefty sum of money for a study that shows their product to be healthful — even if the reporter has to leave out certain facts and slant the evidence.

Our lifestyle often boils down to choosing whom we believe. If we trust physicians and the media more than we do the Heavenly Father, He will leave us to the consequences of our choices. On the other hand, if we put our complete trust in Him, we can claim the promise in Exodus 15:26 for disease avoidance and health restoration.

As far as gallbladder problems go, ignorance isn't always bliss. And some statistics published in the media could stand careful scrutiny. So as milk prices soar, keep your eyes and ears open. Consumers may be "milked" in more ways than one!

11. Baby Food

People who live on milk are like babies who don't really know what is right. Solid food is for mature people who have been trained to know right from wrong. — Hebrews 5:13-14 *Contemporary English Version*© *1995* Copyright by the American Bible Society

Although the above text compares people who take their spiritual nourishment from religious leaders — rather than studying for themselves — to babies who still drink milk because they haven't yet learned to eat solid food, the unspoken health message is that milk is for babies rather than adults.

The Way Things Were

When Yahweh promised in Leviticus 20:24 to lead the Israelites into the land of "milk and honey," they knew the expression meant the land was rich and productive. And some Jewish scholars claim the phrase "milk and honey" assured the Israelites that their nursing mothers would always have enough breast milk for their babies.

The majority of Israelites herded sheep and goats besides growing their own food. They looked forward to Canaan's ideal growing conditions, but depended on goat's milk for supplementing mother's milk. In fact during King Solomon's reign, Yahweh promised them they'd have plenty of GOAT (not COW's) milk for their households and servants if they clung to His covenant and followed His principles. (Proverbs 27:27)

Anyone who's drunk goat milk realizes it doesn't stay fresh long. But fresh milk is best for babies.

Blue Ribbon Baby Food

The best baby milk available has always been Yahweh's personal brand, straight from mother to infant with no middleman.

In the mid-1920s, though, it became fashionable to bottle-feed infants. Even my mother was caught up in the fad for a couple years and bottle-fed my older sister, who suffered all through childhood from both eczema and asthma. Many years later, research showed these ailments can be directly attributed to cow's milk sensitivity and allergies.

By the time I was born, Mom had grown tired of sterilizing bottles and went back to the inexpensive, more health-producing, natural way for nourishing me until my teeth came in. Neither I, nor my other breast-fed siblings, suffered from asthma or eczema.

The Natural Way

When I was nursing my own babies in the 1970s, the health magazines ran several articles about bottle-fed babies' being more susceptible to ear infections than are breast-fed ones. None of my little ones had ear infections before they were weaned; and I mixed their baby cereal with soy milk rather than cow's milk as they adapted to solid foods.

Although I haven't seen as much literature about ear infections in bottle-fed babies lately, I've met a few women who weren't able to nurse their babies, for one reason or another; and had to use baby formula. Some of their children, especially those who drank cow's milk-based formula, have had more than one ear infection.

Down on the Farm

When I was a youngster, Dad tried a number of occupations before he found one he finally liked. In 1945 he bought a small farm with about thirty milking cows, and I often visited the barn to watch the cows being milked. After the milk was collected and pasteurized, most of it was sent to the bottling plant, and Dad kept out enough cream for us to churn our weekly supply of butter and for Mom to whip a topping for Sunday's dessert.

All summer long, our cows ate grass in the same pasture where I picked blueberries. While the cows were being milked, they chomped on oats. When winter came, they ate the baled hay and the silage stored in our silo. They weren't given any chemicals, hormones, or extra protein; and there was no talk of Mad Cow Disease, osteoporosis, or premature puberty in young girls. Breast cancer was rare back then, too.

Tired of farming, Dad soon sold the farm and went into the auction business. Not long after that, dairy farmers began homogenizing milk, but I couldn't stand the taste and quit drinking it plain, although I enjoyed an occasional chocolate or strawberry milkshake. Giving up milk was probably a smart move, though I didn't know it then, because by age twelve I'd already developed a few allergies that could have been caused by the milk and cheese my mother used in cooking.

Speaking of Allergies . . .

Allergies are becoming more prevalent and troublesome in our society. Very rarely is an infant allergic to his own mother's milk, but many have been shown to be allergic to cow's milk and to baby formulas prepared with whey or dried milk powder (*Annals* 1951, *Polish Journal* 1995, and *Pediatrics*-1 1994).

In addition, *The Lancet* has, on more than one occasion, warned its readers that "hypersensitivity to milk is implicated as a cause of sudden death in infancy" (1960 + 1994).

UnChristmas Carol
(Tune: "O Little Town of Bethlehem")

O little town of Death and Phlegm
How still I see thee lie!
Above thy deep and dreamless sleep,
Your children sometimes die.
Clogged noses and congested breath

Are nobody's delight.
Milk chocolate treats and cheesy snacks
Congest thy lungs tonight.
        — Courtesy of the Notmilkman

This next quotation comes out of Palestine: "Dairy products may play a major role in the development of allergies, asthma, sleep difficulties, and migraine headaches" (IJMS 1983). One of my aunts, who drank milk every day because she thought it was good for us, suffered from severe migraine headaches. Her medicine chest was filled with prescription drugs, but none of them ever stopped the migraines. Her doctors were probably so busy prescribing her medications that they didn't have time to read up on the research.

Dr. Mead says, "At least 50% of all children in the United States are allergic to cow's milk, many undiagnosed. Dairy products are the leading cause of food allergy…. Many cases of asthma and sinus infections are reported to be relieved and even eliminated by cutting out dairy" (Mead 1994).

Several journals have reported life-threatening ailments in babies allergic to cow's milk. "Whole casein [milk protein] appears to be highly allergenic . . . 85% of the patients presented response to each of the four caseins" (AAI 1998).

Diabetologia (2001) reported on a Finnish study of 3,000 infants' genes. The researchers' conclusion was this: "Early introduction of cow's milk increased susceptibility to Type I diabetes," an insulin-deficient disease that often strikes young children.

"Milk buffers gastric pH so that food in the stomach ferments and putrefies," causing irritability, mood swings, and depression (Klotter 1994). In addition, the *Polish Journal* reported in 1995 that one year hypersensitivity to milk was "suspected in 62.7 percent of the babies hospitalized with pneumonia or bronchitis."

Moo-less Milk Recipes for Baby

Almond milk has nearly four times the nutrition of cow's milk except for Vitamin B-6. Here's a recipe for almond milk, made in a high speed blender such as a VitaMix®:

Place one cup of soaked almonds (with the skins removed) in the blender with four cups of water. Whiz at highest speed until thoroughly blended. If you don't own a high speed blender, strain the milk through cheese cloth so it'll be thin enough to pass through bottle's nipple. To make up for the missing Vitamin B-6, use a doctor-approved B supplement or add two tablespoons of milk from a young coconut when blending. This makes one quart and will keep in the refrigerator three to five days.

For variety, you can make banana milk with a very ripe banana and one cup distilled water. Other mothers have used cooked white rice, one cup to a quart of water, to break the monotony for baby; but rice milk should have baby vitamins added for best nutrition.

Babies can also thrive on organic soy milk if it doesn't contain too many additives. If they don't like the taste of soy, blend the milk in a high-speed mixer with a pear canned in fruit juice (low sugar).

Years ago, goat milk was considered superior to cow's milk for babies who for some reason couldn't be nursed. But since Mad Cow Disease made its appearance, the plague seems to have affected sheep and goats as well. If I had a baby who couldn't nurse *these days*, I would use one of the above recipes or make a substitute milk using either sunflower seeds, raw cashews, walnuts, or blanched almonds. I've also used seeds and raw nuts in the past to make creamy toppings, delicious dips, and imitation sour cream.

Cow's milk contains at least three substances that cause allergic reactions: lactose [milk sugar], casein [milk protein], and whey [milk plasma]. Whey, the liquid left over after making cheese, contains milk proteins, some minerals, and as much as 75% lactose, depending on the batch. After "factory farming" became the norm, cheese producers began adding the excess whey — left over from the cheese-making process — to other commercial products instead of dumping it.

Some infants outgrow their sensitivity to casein, but many — particularly African Americans — remain lactose intolerant all their lives. These folks suffer from chronic diarrhea, nasal congestion, and Irritable Bowel Syndrome. "Symptoms of milk-protein allergy include cough, choking, gasping, nose colds, asthma, sneezing attacks" (*Annals* 1951).

For those who suffer from asthma and sinus infections, many cases have reported relief "and even elimination" by cutting out dairy (Cohen 2009).

Before we became *complete* vegetarians, when we were still eating dairy products, Frank and I often took the family out for pizza at our favorite restaurant. Pizza was one of my favorites, but I could never eat more than three pieces before I would start gagging. For some reason I never made the connection, but I can remember waking up in the night trying to catch my breath and choking on phlegm following our pizza excursions.

I must have been allergic to casein without knowing it. After giving up pizza and other foods containing dairy products, I realized one day that I no longer experienced those middle-of-the-night episodes.

As a teenager, I was allergic to ragweed and certain pollens too. But after we quit going out for pizza, my hay-fever disappeared as well.

Have You Heard This One?

One of Jerry Seinfeld's comments (to kids): *"Hey, look at those large animals in the field! Let's go squeeze those things underneath them and then drink whatever comes out. Then, let's take whatever's left over, put it aside for a year or so and – eat it!"* Kids: *"Eeeeew!"*

(Courtesy of Robert Cohen)

Zoonoses, as noted in an earlier chapter, can be transmitted through bodily fluids. And milk is one such fluid. Long before the time of Christ, the Egyptians, who had domesticated cattle for both meat and milk, were fairly sure tuberculosis was spread to humans from livestock. Examiners also found evidence of smallpox in Egyptian mummies, including that of Rameses V, and believe the virus was transmitted from cattle (Uic 2011).

Recent studies show that about 75 percent of our newest diseases are of animal origin. One of these is MRSA (methicillin-resistant staphylococcus aureas), which has swept through many American hospitals. A test recorded in the June issue of *Zoonoses Public Health* found MRSA in the milk samples of three dairy herds in Europe (2011). Since the disease is prevalent in our own hospitals, shouldn't we expect the virus that spreads it to be present in our own nation's milk supply as well?

Let's feed our babies the very best milk available, shall we? The protein content helps people sleep better, as we shall see in the next chapter.

12. Milk Allergies and Arthritis

Captain Sisera fled to the tent of Heber, a supposed ally, whose wife Jael offered him a bed and gave him milk to drink. Then, while he was in a deep sleep, she drove a tent peg through his temples and killed him. — Judges 4:17-21 (paraphrased)

The Bible story summarized above doesn't tell us whether Jael drugged the milk before she gave it to Sisera, but it does say he was exhausted and slept soundly. And it's known that a glass of warm milk helps insomniacs fall asleep because of its high protein content. Vegans, on the other hand, often take a cup of warm nut milk or a handful of raw nuts — also high in protein — to help them sleep.

But other than helping someone fall asleep, cow's milk causes more problems than many people realize. The idea that cow's milk belongs in every American adult's diet is a far cry from the truth.

Milk: A Health Food?

Someone nameless, who had a surplus, started a rumor that milk is a *health food*. Those "got milk" ads showing sports stars or beautiful models with milk moustaches were designed to make people think that drinking milk will keep them slim and as healthy-looking as those athletes.

Don't believe those ads! An abundance of research by nonprofit organizations and respected universities shows that cow's milk is NOT a health drink and DOESN'T help you lose weight.

Adults who think they must drink milk for their health should note this: "The enzymes necessary to break down and digest milk are resin and lactase." And in most humans these enzymes are no longer active by age three (Diamond 1985). How can milk be healthful for adults if they have no way to digest it?

We should also think twice when we hear that milk — which is designed to help babies *double* their birth weight — can actually help adults *lose* weight. How cleverly those advertisements hypnotize us into forgetting to use our common sense!

In 1992 the *Journal of Endocrine Reviews* published the work of Clark Grosvenor, who isolated and identified *fifty-nine unique hormones* in every sip of milk. It appears that these hormones are responsible for the big boobs I've seen on some overweight men at the gym lately. Many researchers blame milk products for breast cancer in males and for the early puberty of young American milk-fed girls, too.

Milk is also blamed for acne in adolescents. Although it can be aggravated by stress, acne often clears up when dairy products are eliminated from the diet (Hautarzt 2010). I know mine did. Although I never had acne as bad as some of my school chums, I had a few blackheads once in a while, probably because I was addicted to chocolate candy bars back then. After giving up the candy bars and milkshakes, I was no longer bothered by zits of any color.

We should be leery of any products that are touted as "health foods" if they contain side effects. For instance, red wine has been advocated for digestive ailments and heart problems because it contains flavonoids and antioxidants. But it would be far better to shun the wine, which contains a harmful ingredient (alcohol), and eat the red grapes themselves. Red grapes contain the flavonoids and antioxidants in a purer state than wine because the vitamins, minerals, and enzymes haven't been adulterated.

It's not true, either, that cow's milk is the ONLY food that contains calcium. The calcium in leafy green veggies is much easier for the body to digest and to assimilate than that found in cow's milk. In addition, greens don't contain inorganic hormones and antibiotics that dairy farmers often give their cattle to fatten them and fight various diseases.

Vegans who eat plenty of dark, leafy green vegetables get sufficient calcium. People who decide to switch from cow's milk to a healthier source of calcium should plan to have a huge helping of dark, leafy greens every day, whether in a smoothie, a salad, or a bowl of steamed greens. Other calcium-rich plant foods to include in the diet are sesame seeds, organic tofu, raw almonds or Brazil nuts, and flax seeds which are also high in omega-3 fatty acids.

Researchers have discovered that Type 1 Diabetes (insulin-dependent) and multiple sclerosis look almost alike immunologically, in a test tube. The *Journal of Immunology* (April 2001) reported many similarities in the two diseases and has attributed "exposure to cow milk protein as a risk factor in the development of both diseases for people who are genetically susceptible."

At least two different studies have associated the prevalence of MS (multiple sclerosis) with eating dairy foods such as cow's milk, butter, and cream (NRE 1992 and Lindner 2011).

A Brazilian pediatric journal (JP 2007) reported that "the dietary factors which were most responsible for risk of anemia were a greater proportion of calories from cow's milk." It's sad that those who control the media aren't interested in *professional* research because "many studies blame anemia on the consumption of milk and dairy products" (Cohen 2011).

Choose Your Poison

Dr. Honglei Chen, an expert on diet and Parkinson's disease, led a 2007 study of over 100,000 adults, and the findings were published in the *American Journal of Epidemiology*. They found that "milk was positively associated with" Parkinson's (NHD 2011). Whether it was from the pesticides in milk or the higher levels of uric acid that dairy products produce in the body, they weren't sure. But the correlation was unmistakable.

Besides depleting calcium in our bones, cow's milk has also been linked to ovarian cysts and high blood pressure (*Epidemiology* 2009). The same journal also reported a fourteen-year study of Finnish male smokers, including 26,500 who had never had a stroke, and concluded that "intakes of certain dairy foods [including yogurt] may be associated with risk of strokes."

Finally, in addition to allergic symptoms, which often don't show up until the next day, dairy consumption has been blamed (Klotter 1995) for "mood swings, depression, and irritability."

But the most serious problem I myself have experienced from dairy products has been arthritis.

Oh, My Aching Thumbs!

In my twenties I became a vegetarian but still ate dairy products believing, as many do, that I would suffer a protein deficiency if I didn't use cheese and eggs. After Frank's heart attack, we stopped using eggs, but continued buying margarine, ice cream, and cheese. By the time I was in my late forties, however, I had arthritis in both thumbs. The pain was so intense; I was in agony just carrying my briefcase.

Around 1994, when we heard the first reported case of Mad Cow Disease, Frank and I decided we could do without anything that came from an animal. That's when we gave up pizza, and my hay fever went away, as mentioned earlier.

We stopped buying dairy products, and I learned to make simpler meals without milk and cheese. About six months later I noticed my thumbs no longer ached when I carried my briefcase. Many researchers have found a definite connection between arthritis and dairy products. Note these two reports:

"In the case of eight-year-old female subject, juvenile rheumatoid arthritis was a milk allergy. After avoiding dairy products, all pain was gone in three weeks" (JRSM 1985).

A forty-two-year old woman experienced relief of knee pain after eliminating dairy products (Twogood 1991). "Once, after drinking a glass of milk, her knees swelled within twenty minutes."

Ted's physician knew these facts, but he couldn't convince his patient:

That Nosy, Interfering Doctor!

"What did he say?" I asked when Ted came limping out of his doctor's office.

"No doctor is going to tell me what I should or shouldn't eat!" he sputtered. I learned later that his doctor told him his

132

arthritis would probably keep getting worse if he didn't give up the glass of milk with each meal and his nightly dish of ice cream.

What a shame! Ted paid the doctor to give him medical advice, and then he became angry when the doctor did what he was paid to do! What Ted really wanted was a quick fix — with a medicine that would enable him to keep eating the very foods that were making his arthritis worse.

Ted's arthritis got worse after he retired and stopped being active. His legs suffered the most, especially one knee. He started off with a cane, then needed a walker, and finally ended up in a nursing home — enduring much leg pain as he gradually lost the ability to get around. I often wondered if his arthritis would have disappeared, like mine did, if only he'd taken his doctor's advice.

The Bible says, *"Narrow is the way that leads to life and wide is the way that leads to destruction"* (Matthew 7:13+14 paraphrased); but I found a quote by Gene Hicks, quoted in the Nov.-Dec. 2010 *Hope International Newsletter*, that really describes some of our eating habits: *"Narrow is the mind, and wide is the mouth that leads to destruction."*

Delayed Reaction

Some people believe they can tolerate cow's milk only in the form of ice cream. What they don't realize is that icy cold foods neutralize stomach acid and slow down the digestion process, so the problems caused by the milk and sugar don't show up until many hours later. By the time the disturbances appear, most have forgotten what they ate the day before, so they don't make the connection.

Those readers old enough to remember former President John Kennedy (JFK) may recall his back ailment. First he sustained a back injury, and then arthritis set in. His pain was so intense; he often gave televised presidential speeches from his rocking chair, lending an aura of intimacy while hiding his excruciating back pain.

According to one source, JFK wore a full body back brace; and his pain was so severe that he couldn't bend over to tie his own shoes. An article by a White House insider said Kennedy's favorite lunch was grilled cheese sandwiches with a glass of milk. Hmmm. We don't need to be scientists to see the connection between dairy products and his arthritic pain, do we?

Painless, No-Wheeze Pizza

Here's a recipe for a healthier pizza without dairy and the four white poisons:

Place whole-wheat pita bread circles on a cookie sheet and spread with tomato sauce (check label to make sure the sauce contains no cheese). Sprinkle with basil, oregano, or other herbs of choice. Top with chopped onion, pepper slices, and ripe olives, if desired. Across top, sprinkle shredded veggie cheese (from the health-food aisle). Bake at 350 degrees Fahrenheit for about 20 minutes or until cheese melts.

Note: For a less expensive, healthful cheese substitute, search for a vegan cheese recipe online. Many blogs and

134

websites contain home-made cheese recipes for people wanting to cut out dairy and packaged foods.

This statement has been attributed to famous author James Joyce: *"A corpse is meat gone bad. Well and what's cheese? Corpse of milk."*

Aged cheese contains *tyramine*, a substance that is believed to damage the frontal lobe of the brain.

Additionally, cheese has been blamed for many hormone problems. Poor semen quality in some men has been attributed to a diet rich in cheese. Put a husband who eats cheese every day in bed with a wife who has adrenal problems from low-blood-sugar, and the stage is set for infertility, hormone imbalances, post-partum anxiety, and depression.

It's time we weaned ourselves from milk and adopted an adult diet. And while we're at it, let's look at the osteoporosis scare as well.

13. Osteoporosis

Beware of false prophets, which come to you in sheep's clothing, but inwardly they are ravening wolves. — Matthew 7:13

We've heard of false prophets in the spiritual realm, but what about the medical field? Is it possible that vendors touting their wares might scare us into buying products we don't really need?

Milking the Public

Sometime during the twentieth century, somebody started a rumor that you need to drink milk to have strong bones. That lie has been perpetrated by wise marketers who began losing money when the public learned about *factory farming* and has been perpetuated by media reports based on tainted studies paid for by certain special interest groups.

Have you been following the statistics about osteoporosis? In 1993 the June *Nutrition Action Health Letter*

[NAHL] reported that countries "with the highest rates of osteoporosis, such as the United States, England, and Sweden, consume the most milk. China and Japan, where people eat much less animal protein and dairy food, have low rates of osteoporosis." And recent reports show that in areas where these people are adopting a more Western style diet, their rate of osteoporosis is rising.

Statistics show that milk drinking does nothing to prevent osteoporosis. In fact, the opposite is true.

Many physicians report learning hardly anything about nutrition in medical school. And when they finish their education they're too busy, setting up their practices and paying off their college loans, to read all the available literature. Most of them consider themselves lucky if they can keep up with the research in their own area of specialization.

There are, however, a few doctors who've discovered that cow's milk isn't the miracle food it's touted to be. Most of them agree that dairy products cause more harm than good. The Notmilkman alerted me to the following *voices crying in the wilderness*:

"The commercials do not point out . . . that osteoporosis is common among milk drinkers" (Dr. Neal Barnard).

"Milk . . . is not the solution to poor bone density. To the contrary, it's part of the problem" (Dr. Charles Attwood).

These anti-dairy prophets agree with the findings of the China Study (Campbells 2006): "The association between the intake of animal protein and fracture rates appears to be as strong as the association between cigarette smoking and lung cancer."

No Bones about It!

Of the 250,000 people with bone disease in Africa, most are from the Massa tribe whose diet consists of blood and cow's milk. And in America, most of the 30 million people with bone disease partake heavily of milk or ice cream or both.

A number of researchers have reported that when the diet is high in animal protein, our bodies must leach calcium from our bones in order to neutralize the acid condition caused by the protein overload. A Japanese study showed "calcium intake demonstrated no protective [element] in preventing bone fractures. In fact, those populations with the highest calcium intakes had higher fracture rates than those with more modest calcium intakes" (Calif Tissue Int 1992). Also, "Increasing one's protein intake by 100% may cause calcium loss to double" (AJCN 1981). Like the previous one, this last study was referring to animal protein, not plant protein.

While reporting in 1988 that the "average man in the U.S. eats 175% more protein than the recommended daily allowance, and the average woman eats 144% more," the U.S. Surgeon General issued a public health warning. Quoting a scientific journal (SciM 1986), he declared that "osteoporosis is caused by a number of things, one of the most important being too much dietary protein." This study, like the previous ones, was referring to *animal* protein.

Double Robbery

One of the biggest myths propagated in America is that, if you don't drink milk, you need to take calcium supplements or a prescription drug to avoid osteoporosis, a skeletal disorder in which the bones become extremely porous and are subject to fracture due to low bone mineral density. However, the research shows something entirely different.

"Even when eating 1,400 mg. of calcium daily, one can lose up to 4% of his or her bone mass each year while consuming a high-protein diet" (AJCN 1979). That's because the real culprit is excess animal protein, and not a lack of calcium-rich foods.

The Physicians Committee for Responsible Medicine reports, "You can decrease your risk of osteoporosis by reducing sodium and animal protein intake in the diet" as well as exercising and increasing your intake of fruits and vegetables — especially kale, broccoli, leafy green veggies, and beans (Physicians 2007).

If you want to get enough calcium, eat plenty of cooked Chinese cabbage, spinach, kale, bok choy, broccoli, rhubarb, and beans, including pinto, white, and red ones. Don't eat a *dog food* diet (same foods, day in and day out). Vary your choices, eating different greens and beans throughout the week.

According to Goldschmidt, about 87 percent of women may have been incorrectly diagnosed as having osteoporosis because a Mayo Clinic College of Medicine study showed that "only 13 to 18 percent of women older than 50 meet the correct diagnosis for osteoporosis" (Goldschmidt 2010).

Getting plenty of variety in your choice of salads and cooked veggies may keep you out of both camps — those with osteoporosis and those who have some other ailment that mimics the disease.

If you're concerned about osteoporosis, the following culprits have also been implicated, according to some nutritionists:

-- Overuse of table salt
-- Food preservatives and additives
-- Excess sugar in the diet
-- Soft drinks
-- Excess fluoride in the system
-- Mercury poisoning (from ingesting toxic fish and/or from leaky amalgam fillings)

When I became a vegetarian, I started buying soymilk for cooking and for pouring over our breakfast cereal. I also gave it to my children after they were weaned. This was many years before someone started the rumor that soy beans are poisonous and should be avoided at all costs. My oldest is almost fifty, and none of my children have yet suffered from soy bean poisoning.

Actually, fresh green soy beans are not only healthful, but they're delicious steamed, even without butter and salt! Not only that, but they contain all the essential amino acids.

Women who eat tofu or drink soymilk regularly have been found to go through menopause with much less difficulty, and to suffer from fewer hot flashes, than women who eat meat and dairy. The same has been said of vegan women who stick to a low-fat diet (JCO 2008). Organic tofu and soymilk are healthful if they're not processed to death or filled with unhealthy additives, such as MSG and carrageenan.

Soy Bashers

Soy beans have been blamed for many ailments, though. And there's a little truth mixed in with the lie. Soy foods — like meat analogs and other commercial products containing soy isolate, soy protein, and isoflavones — are not "whole" foods. And they're super-high in refined soy protein. Yahweh never intended us to remove all the protein from a particular food and then add large concentrates of it to any other food.

People who eat largely of soy-meat analogs and other foods containing soy isolates, rather than the whole soy bean, place a heavy burden on their thyroid gland. These people start feeling tired early in the day, tend to gain unwanted pounds, and have trouble staying awake during the afternoon. Frank was having all these symptoms a few years ago. Convinced that his beloved "veggie meats" (made with soy isolates) were the cause, he stopped eating them for a few weeks. To his surprise, all those symptoms disappeared. Instead of meat analogs; he now enjoys my homemade oatmeal burgers — no more worries about MSG, carrageenan, or chemical additives.

Eat green organic soy beans, like any other garden vegetable, when they haven't been processed to death or adulterated with lots of additives. They're much better for your bones than a glass of cow's milk! In addition, the *Journal of Clinical Oncology* (JCO 2008) reported that "women who consume soy products have a lower risk of breast cancer than women who do not eat soy."

Estrogen vs. Phytoestrogens

Don't confuse the estrogen in cow's milk and hormone supplements with the phytoestrogens in soy beans. *Phyto* means "plant," and *phytoestrogens* are estrogen disrupters. The *human estrogen hormone* is a steroid, and has been implicated in breast cancer, whereas plant estrogens are healthful nutrients.

In fact, July 2011's *Journal of Membrane Biology* reported on the results of a study showing that *genestein*, the phytoestrogen found in soy, actually disrupts the spreading of cancer cells. These findings have been duplicated by the Shanghai University Medical School which concluded (AJCN 11/11): "Our findings indicate that the consumption of soy food is associated with lower lung cancer risk."

So the next time a soy basher tells you soy beans are poisonous, tell them that apples, brown rice, and broccoli all contain the same kinds of phytoestrogens found in green soy beans. You may eat them without guilt or fear of being poisoned. On the other hand, if you fill up on meat analogs containing soy protein or isolates, you may indeed find yourself suffering from protein poisoning!

As Dr. John McDougall says, "Eating a high protein diet is like pouring acid rain on your bones" (AD 2010).

Vitamin D Upgrade

Dr. Gominak (2011) says osteoporosis is really caused by low amounts of Vitamin D, rather than from a lack of calcium. So let's go there for a minute.

In grade school they taught us that Vitamin D is the "sunshine vitamin." Now, though, nutritionists claim it shouldn't really be called a vitamin at all, since it's actually a hormone. We get vitamins from the foods we eat, but hormones aren't found in food (unless they're added to animals' diets, to make them grow quicker). Hormones are usually produced in our own bodies (Gominak 2011).

As mentioned earlier, hormone D is produced just underneath our skin, where our GOOD cholesterol transforms ultraviolet rays into this steroid (previously called Vitamin D) that prevents rickets. Symptoms of rickets include skeletal deformities such as bowed legs, abnormally curved spine, thickened wrists and ankles, and breastbone projection (Mayo 2011).

Defective Receptors

In otherwise healthy people, ten to fifteen minutes of sunlight, two or three times a week, will ensure proper hormone D levels (IADM 2008). However, in countries where women must be veiled whenever they go out in public, their faces and arms don't receive adequate sunlight, even though they live in the sunniest areas of our continent. These individuals must try to get their hormone D from supplements, as do liver or kidney patients with defective D receptors which can't transform the sunlight into this usable hormone (Vivo 2012).

I'm wondering if the reason so many Americans are deficient in Vitamin D is because they're actually in Stage One of kidney failure and don't know it. Their D receptors may not be working at peak efficiency, like the receptors of the liver and kidney patients mentioned earlier.

In addition to osteoporosis, Dr. Gominak (2011) believes that low amounts of Hormone D (found in patients suffering from autoimmune diseases, sleep disorders and kidney stones) and the increase in breast, colon, and prostate cancers are contributors to those conditions.

Have You Seen My D?

Since breast milk contains no hormone D, new mothers are urged to get outdoors with their little ones on sunny days. Women who've had a few close–together pregnancies are also at risk of having low D levels since the body doesn't store the reserves during pregnancy.

According to Dr. Lipman (2012), Vitamin D is the "most potent steroid hormone" in the body. He also claims that sun exposure is the best possible way to get the needed hormone and that we can get only ten percent of the amount needed from fortified foods.

Just a reminder: Sunburns, although painful, may be a cause of skin cancer; but they don't cause Vitamin D toxicity. Overdosing on supplements is the only cause!

Precautions with D Supplements

For that reason, many who take D need to be under a practitioner's care. In choosing a supplement, many vegetarians swear by Vitamin D-3, which is advertised as "vegetarian." However, *calciferol*, the supposedly vegetable ingredient in D-3, comes from lanolin. Lanolin comes from lamb's wool, and sheep are NOT *vegetables*.

In addition, since Vitamin D is a steroid, people who've had heart problems may suffer chest pains as a side effect and should get expert advice when taking it in supplement form.

Since D-3 is toxic in overdose, seek professional advice before taking large amounts of this hormone. *New England Journal of Medicine* reported that "Hypervitaminosis D may result from drinking milk that is incorrectly and excessively fortified with vitamin D." People drinking D-fortified milk should be carefully monitored (NEJM 1992).

Anyone taking 5,000 IU daily should have a spot blood test every three months; and those taking 10,000 IU per day should have their calcium-phosphorus-parathyroid levels tested every three months as well.

Apparently it doesn't take much! "Consuming as little as 45 micrograms of Vitamin D-3 in young children has resulted in signs of overdose" (*Pediatrics-2* 1963). It's not just in children, either. The *Canadian Medical Association Journal* (1992) also warned about excess Vitamin D intake in adults. It "increases aluminum absorption, and high aluminum levels in the body may cause an Alzheimer's-like disease."

If an overdose is toxic in both children and adults, imagine the amount ingested by people who drink large amounts of cow's milk fortified with D!

Now let's look at a couple of Bible texts that have baffled people for years.

14. Time Out

Women who have recently borne a son shall avoid crowds for 40 days; and if they bear a daughter, they shall stay away from the synagogue and other public places for 80 days. — Leviticus 12:1-5 (paraphrased)

The above command stumped Dennis and Brenda Kaneshiro, who wanted to obey all Yahweh's statutes and judgments. Deeply interested in natural medicine, they asked a physician-friend if he could give them a medical reason for the two varying recovery periods. The only suggestion the doctor could think of was that a woman's immune system is depressed during pregnancy, to keep the white blood cells from seeing the fetus as a "foreign intruder" and attacking it.

This aroused their curiosity, and they checked Brenda's blood after her deliveries. After the birth of their son, it took forty days for her white blood-cell count to return to normal. When they checked Brenda's blood forty days after their *daughter's* birth, though, it contained very few white blood cells. Guess when her blood count registered a healthy number? That's right — the 80th day!

They decided a pregnant woman's body must recognize a female-fetus as more of an intruder and a threat to the mother's immune system than does a male one. Apparently Yahweh arranged for the woman's immune system to shut down even more, for the embryo's protection, while a mother is carrying a female baby.

By the way, it once bothered me that when I'd go to obstetricians for a pre-natal exam, they would invariably write "pregnancy" on the medical form where it asked the patient's illness. At the time, I believed pregnancy was just a normal occurrence. But now that I know a woman's immune system is suppressed during pregnancy, it makes sense to classify the condition as an illness.

And just as a baby boy's blood absolutely clots best for circumcision on his eighth day of life, so women who adhere to the quarantine period prescribed in Leviticus 12 are less apt to catch a cold or other contagious disease when they attend public gatherings with their new babies.

Contrary to the belief that this principle was a punishment for women who bore a girl-child rather than a male one, the precept shows Yahweh's love for all His children by giving guidelines for a mother's full recovery after the childbirth process.

.

The separation of lepers from the rest of society eventually came to be seen as a punishment for being *unclean*. But quarantine, according to Yahweh, wasn't as much a moral precept as it was a protection. Substitute the word *contagious* for the word *unclean* and remember how quarantine periods saved many children from measles, mumps, smallpox and chicken pox before there were vaccinations, and from scarlet fever as well.

In fact, disease containment was the original purpose for leper colonies. And while trying to find a cure for leprosy, medical authorities discovered that both kinds of leprosy — the one that begins as skin lesions and the one that first affects the mucus membranes, though they both result in the same disabilities later on — are spread through bodily fluids.

Now that they've found a drug that seems to work, Norwegian authorities no longer demand quarantine for lepers. And they've changed the name to Hansen's disease to decrease the stigma and prevent panicking.

But quarantine is still an effective disease controller, especially in SARS, the *severe acute respiratory syndrome* that threatened to become a world-wide epidemic a few years ago. Like leprosy, SARS is spread by a virus contained in bodily liquids and can travel through the air when the infected person coughs or sneezes.

Sanitation

During the bubonic plague, people were dying right and left. Only the wealthy, who could afford to escape to the countryside where the air was cleaner, were spared. But doctors eventually stumbled on the Bible prescription for curtailing the spread of typhoid, cholera, and dysentery. Yahweh's instruction in Deut. 23:12 and 13, to cover one's excrement, isn't merely a guideline for keeping the air smelling sweet. Covering sewage and other waste products also cuts down the number of air-borne vermin who feed on excrement and garbage and, thus, spread germs wherever they go.

Hidden Health Hazard

The story is often told of Dr. Semmelweis in Vienna, who was alarmed at the rate of women's deaths in the hospital's obstetrics ward in the late 1840's. He noticed that the medical students walked from their morning classes in the mortuary, where they performed autopsies, directly to the women's ward where they practiced giving vaginal exams. One in every six new mothers hospitalized there died of sepsis fever. After he commanded the students to wash their hands before entering the women's ward, the death rate among these new mothers dropped drastically.

Unfortunately, the medical students complained to the hospital authorities, and Semmelweis wasn't allowed to stay and "hinder" the hospital's work. Leaving Vienna, he went to

Budapest, where he had the same success in cutting the death rate of new mothers in the hospital there. But again, he was censored and left in disrespect. Many years later his findings were found to be life-saving, and hand-washing became standard hospital procedure; but Semmelweis was never honored for his discovery.

Whether or not he realized it, Semmelweis had stumbled upon one of Yahweh's health precepts in Numbers 19 — that touching dead bodies or the blood from sick and dying animals is a health hazard. The Bible instructs us to wash in clean water after coming in contact with a corpse. The charcoal water filters in use today may be a carryover from the days when the Israelites were instructed to put ashes — ground charcoal — in their "water of purification" (found in Numbers 19:11-12).

If time lasts long enough, researchers will probably find valid medical reasons for every single precept Yahweh gave in His *torah*.

That goes for healthy hearts too. Read on . . . .

15. Heartaches

Keep thy heart with all diligence; for out of it are the issues of life.   — Proverbs 4:23

What are the *issues* that flow from our hearts? Blood! Some modern Bible versions use the word *source* instead of *issues*. And Yahweh tells us "the life is in the blood." Our heart is busy pumping blood day and night, and Yahweh cautions us to take care of it — not just in the spiritual realm, but also in the physical.

Most of us know we shouldn't exercise strenuously after a heavy meal. But that fact wasn't well known in the early 1970s when our town's high school coach went down to his basement to exercise after eating a big Thanksgiving dinner. He died that night, leaving behind his wife and three young children.

The Bible warns us against overeating (i.e., being a "glutton"); and it's a terrific strain on the heart if we also exercise strenuously after doing so. One of our neighbor-friends apparently hadn't heard the news. Her husband was outdoors shoveling one morning, after a heavy snowfall, and she was worried that he was working too hard. When he came in for a drink of water and to catch his breath, she insisted he sit down to a meal of pancakes. And she kept piling more food on his plate, thinking the more he ate, the more rest he'd get before he went back outside.

After he went back outdoors and resumed shoveling the snow, though, he suffered a massive heart attack and died right there in the driveway. If she'd known that our hearts cannot handle the work involved in food digestion AND strenuous exercise at the same time, her husband might still be alive.

Heart Attacks on the Increase

A 2011 news article reported that, according to the American Heart Association, nearly one third of all Americans have some sort of heart disease. Their statistics showed that one of every six deaths in the U.S. is the result of heart attack or angina (heart disease). Over 1.25 million heart attacks occur each year, and an estimated 10 million Americans suffer from angina.

Different Perspectives

Incidentally, a study by Dr. Hanna Gardner in Miami showed "a 61 percent higher incidence of heart disease in people who drank soda each day" than in those who drank no soda at all. Her study (Gardner 2011) showed no difference "whether it was diet soda or regular." That report surprised me because many cardiologists tell their heart patients to cut down on red meats, but they don't usually mention soda pop.

Heart disease, otherwise known as angina, results from inflammation in the arteries, caused by homocysteine, or acid waste. Vitamin B breaks down this acid waste so we can eliminate wastes from our bodies by way of perspiration or bowel movements. However, if we have a deficiency of the B vitamins, the homocysteine causes a plaque build-up in our arteries, increasing our heart attack risk by 300 percent. One way to keep a high level of the B vitamins in our bodies is to eat plenty of leafy greens and veggies; but overeaters usually tend to indulge in acid-producing foods rather than the vitamin-rich ones.

Some people with angina go in for bypass surgery. Studies, though, show that having a stent inserted is like bandaging an open wound that won't stop bleeding. If the person doesn't change her lifestyle, she'll soon need another stent.

Heart disease is "basically a terminal disease," says Dr. Katz (Katz 2010). "All the heart bypasses and arterial stents in the world . . . on their own do not solve the problem."

While heart disease often makes itself known gradually, the same isn't true of heart attacks not related to angina. Some people have no warning that their heart is impaired. Frank was one of those people. His heart attack struck unexpectedly.

Frank's Heart Attack

Before Frank had his heart attack, he thought he was safe, because he didn't eat meat. The literature all said that saturated fat and cholesterol cause plaque build-up in the arteries, narrowing them and making it hard for the blood platelets to pass through them. Since he knew the bad cholesterol (LDL) comes from animal fat, he — as a vegetarian — believed he was not at risk.

And when he was admitted to the hospital, they didn't find a blocked artery. Although the results showed an inferior heart attack, in which a portion of the heart dies, the only abnormalities they could find were in a blood sample: his triglyceride count was extremely high.

Triglycerides accumulate when we eat a lot of rich food, including desserts. Because we had five children to feed, Frank often brought home a carload of fancy breads and high-fat pastries from a thrift bakery, and we purchased our soybean oil — which I used freely in those days — in large jugs at a discount store. Also, one of our sons worked at a chicken factory at the time and could bring home a flat of five-dozen eggs whenever he wanted.

"Eggs are higher in cholesterol than any other food, making them a contributor to cardiovascular disease" (Vegan 2010). Frank had lots of time to think about his eating habits while he lay in the hospital, and after he was released he told me he'd often fried himself a dozen eggs at a time whenever I took the children somewhere and wasn't home to see what he was doing. In his hospital bed, he determined that he'd rather live without eggs than die over them. He hasn't fried an egg since.

Who's Who?

By the way, all the case histories in this book are true. Frank has given me permission to share his medical miseries and the lessons we've learned, hoping they will keep someone else from making the same mistakes. I know my father would feel the same way if he were still alive. Some of our friends have also consented to have their stories told; but I've changed the names of people I couldn't reach, to avoid embarrassing them or their families.

Other Factors

Another contributor to heart attacks is overwork. A study published in *Annals of Internal Medicine* found that those who work more than eleven hours a day are 67 percent more likely to have a heart attack than those who work an eight-hour day (Borland 2011). And overwork may have been a factor in Frank's case, too, because he tried to clear a whole field of small trees with his chain saw the day before his heart attack.

Frank has a mellow baritone voice, and — when we were first married —we often sang duets together; but since his heart attack in 1981 he hasn't been able to get through a whole song without running out of steam.

Frank took heart medicine for several years, but finally decided it was a "crutch" and weaned himself off all medication in 1988. His heart has been fine ever since. Even today, though, if we're in room where people are smoking, he has trouble breathing.

Arterial Plaque

In the 1960s doctors in Africa didn't know what a "bad" heart looked like. Heart attacks were on the rise here in America, so African doctors would send to America requesting some autopsied hearts to show their medical students. At the time, Americans ate more fatty meats and fast food than people in Africa. But since many Africans have adopted a Western diet, their teachers no longer order autopsied hearts and blocked arteries from America for their medical schools. They have their own African specimens now.

Britain's War Story

During World War II, people all over Britain planted "victory gardens" because meat was scarce and many foods were rationed. While the people worked their gardens and ate home-grown produce, the rate of heart attacks dropped considerably. This stymied the doctors, who assumed people would have more heart attacks during a war, simply from the stress of bombings, air raids, and fears of being attacked.

After the war, many people gave up their gardens when food-rationing ended. Peace reigned, but the rate of heart attacks rose. Research started bringing to light the knowledge of cholesterol and saturated-fat buildup in the arteries. Anyone who paid attention to the nightly news or read the newspaper in the late 1960s and early 1970s heard the warnings about cutting down on meat.

Britain's experience agrees with an AJE article published in 1995, reporting that "vegetarian diets have been successful in arresting coronary artery [heart-related] disease." And JAMA's article, published the same year, claimed that a vegetarian diet actually *reversed* heart disease!

But diet isn't the only factor in heart disease. Brian Tracy (Tracy 1995) claims, "Outbursts of anger can cause heart attacks, strokes, burst blood vessels, ulcers, migraine headaches, asthma, and skin diseases of all kinds."

Where did he get that idea?

What the Doctor Said

When he sent Frank home from the hospital, the doctor didn't prescribe a special diet. His only precaution was this: "Unless you want another heart attack, DO NOT GET ANGRY!"

That surprised Frank, but he wanted to live to see his children grow up. Giving up fried eggs would be easy, though, compared to taking his doctor's advice. Quick to blow up at a moment's notice, he knew he'd have to change his whole attitude. With lots of prayer, he found other ways to handle upsets and is still alive thirty-plus years later.

Where did the doctor get the advice he gave Frank? Had he read the following passage?

Be ye angry, and sin not; let not the sun
go down upon your wrath; Neither give
place to the devil. — Ephesians 4:26-27

An Ohio State University study (Mental 2011) found that "those who had less control over their anger tended to heal more slowly from wounds," that people whose anger is easily aroused and then harbored "cause significant and cumulative damage to their bodies," and that men who don't manage their anger well are "more likely to suffer a heart attack before age 55 than their more emotionally controlled peers."

Harvard University has published several studies with the following findings: (1) outbursts of anger double a person's risk of having a heart attack, (2) one in every 40 heart attack survivors reported an "episode of anger" in the two hours before their attack, and (3) in people who've already had one heart attack, an episode of anger raises their risk of having another heart attack by 200 percent (Smart-heart 2011).

After reading the first draft of this book, my friend Ruth remembered one of her former patients: "He sat up in bed, screamed at his grown children who were gathered around his hospital bed, and fell back dead of a heart attack," she told me.

According to the Scriptures, anger is NOT a sin; it's what we *do* with the anger that's the problem. Do we keep the anger inside and let it fester until it attacks our blood vessels?

Years ago, a pastor told me he took a walk whenever he got angry. Just getting out in the fresh air did something to calm his nerves, and the exercise was good for his heart at the same time. Some men go to their workshop and pound nails, turning their anger into creativity.

Do our outbursts hurt anybody else? Some people get angry at their spouse and kick the cat. Others get angry at the cat and kick their spouse. Neither reaction is a responsible way to release anger.

Frank's friend Bruce has a wonderful technique for dealing with his anger. I often feel threatened when some "so-called adults" throw temper tantrums, but I'm not threatened when I watch Bruce vent his anger. He pounds his fist into his open palm and shouts, "I'm angry!" several times. After a few outbursts, he feels good again, and no one has been hurt in the process.

Bad Hat = Bad Heart

As stated previously, anger is a natural human emotion. But we need to learn positive ways to manage it — if we want to stay healthy. The story of Nabal, an Israelite whom the Bible describes as *churlish*, shows what can happen to bad-tempered people.

According to the story, when David was fleeing from King Saul, he sent some of his men to beg food from Nabal, a rich landowner. David and his men had been living in this man's fields, protecting his livestock and crops from predators and wild animals. But the ungrateful Nabal snarled at the men and sent them away empty-handed.

When David heard about the man's ingratitude, he became angry and prepared to take revenge by attacking Nabal's household. But Nabal's servants had overheard their master's angry tirade and alerted his wife Abigail, who intercepted David and his men with an abundance of food and an apology for her husband's inhospitable behavior. While presenting the food, she talked David out of his anger and persuaded him not to take any action he might later regret.

David wisely listened to her good judgment, accepted the food, and let his anger subside. But when Abigail later told her husband how she'd intercepted David and his men and saved the family and their property from destruction, the Bible says Nabal's "heart died within him, and he became as a stone."

Nabal's plight sounds like a description of a heart attack and a stroke, occurring at the same time, doesn't it? Whatever the medical description, Nabal was comatose when he died ten days later. The complete story is in First Samuel, Chapter 25.

Surely the churning of milk bringeth forth butter, and the wringing of the nose bringeth forth blood: so the forcing of wrath [anger] bringeth forth strife. — Proverbs 30:33

Whatever we do, we shouldn't act rashly like the Spec 4 who got angry at his first sergeant. Frank often tells this story, which occurred while he was in the Army, working in a medical dispensary. The two other men were all alone in the barracks while everyone else had gone out partying. They had their own bottles of booze, and as they were drinking companionably, they got into an argument.

The more they drank, the more they disagreed, and the Spec 4 finally lost control. In a rage, he pulled out his knife and stabbed the sergeant, cutting him from one kidney to the other. Fortunately, they weren't far from the medical dispensary, and the medics were able to save the sergeant. But the Spec 4 was court-martialed and sent to Federal Prison.

The Biblical principle – that "fostered" anger brings forth strife – was certainly true in this instance. Some people drink alcohol ONLY when they get upset, but that can lead to personal health problems, as well.

16. Fatal Choices

It is not for kings to drink wine; nor for princes strong drink: Lest they drink, and forget the law, and pervert the judgment of any of the afflicted.
— Proverbs 31:4-5

Long before Christ was born, two young priests under the influence of alcohol thought Yahweh wouldn't mind if they lit their censors with a different flame from the one He'd consecrated. After He sent fire from heaven and destroyed them, Yahweh commanded that priests weren't to drink wine or any other fermented drinks while they were on duty. This story appears in Leviticus 10:1-10.

Back then, the priests all came from the tribe of Levi. And the sons of Aaron were dedicated from birth to serve Yahweh. But if men from a different tribe wanted to dedicate themselves to the Lord's service or build a closer walk with God for a certain length of time, they were allowed to take the "Nazarite" vow. While performing this vow, the men let their hair grow long as a reminder of their decision. During this time they were not only prohibited from drinking wine, but they were not even allowed to eat grapes until their period of consecration ended, at which time they cut their hair as a public announcement that they'd completed their vow.

But it's not only Yahweh's priests and people taking a vow who are warned not to ingest alcohol. King Solomon, in the Book of Proverbs, wrote that kings and rulers (people in responsible, decision-making positions) shouldn't drink wine, nor should they even ASK for a strong drink. And in the New Testament, Peter warns all of us (followers of Christ) to be *sober*. A study on the original meaning of the word *sober* shows that it means to "abstain from harmful substances."

> *Wine makes men foolish, and strong drink makes*
> *men come to blows; and whoever comes into error*
> *through these is not wise.*
> —Proverbs 20:1, *Bible in Basic English*

As a medic in the Army, Frank can testify to the truth in the above verse.

Frank's War Stories

Most of the villagers near Frank's overseas Army base were communists, and they didn't like Americans because of the trouble our men often caused in their town. So the following incident shouldn't be too surprising:

One very quiet young enlisted man was usually shy around women. Apparently a few drinks would loosen him up, though. One night he went downtown and, after a few drinks, suddenly got brave enough to approach the women in the bar. There was enough snow on the ground for snowballs, and he had the *not-so-brilliant* idea of putting snowballs down the necks of the women's dresses.

Frank doesn't know how many attempts the man got away with before he chose the wrong young woman – one with a boyfriend. The boyfriend hit the enlisted man in the face with a wine bottle, and a bunch of civilians from a nearby table joined the fray. The young man came staggering back to the base, his face cut from his lip to his ear. Frank was on duty when the man came in and had to attend to him. Eventually, the young man's stitches healed, but his face was probably scarred for life.

Another young man was scheduled to be discharged the following Monday and return to the states to get married. But on Sunday night, his friends took him downtown to give him a bachelors' party. After a night of drinking, he somehow smashed his car into a stone wall on the way back to the base. When they brought the man in to the dispensary, Frank didn't recognize him because his face was all ripped apart. In fact, the young man had to be taken to a larger facility where they could attend to all his breaks and wounds. Needless to say, that man didn't return stateside the next day, after all, because he was hospitalized for several weeks. The wedding ceremony – if it ever took place – certainly had to be rescheduled.

More War Stories

Speaking of getting beaten up, Frank met an enlisted man who'd been a cook back in the states. The military base sponsored a "happy hour" for the men, during which time they could order — for a nickel apiece — as many drinks as they wanted. Occasionally this cook would buy twenty shots and put them on the table in front of him, drinking one at a time. After a few drinks, though, he usually got angry at something and began throwing the empty glasses. The MPs arrived on the scene, beat him, and then dragged him to jail. It happened more than once, and the man never seemed to learn his lesson.

Another soldier, highly decorated after World War II, had re-enlisted and was in Frank's unit. But this man had a drinking problem and couldn't keep his promotions. Every so often he'd drink too much, trash an area of the barracks and get demoted. No sooner would he get his stripes back than he'd go out drinking, to celebrate, and lose them again for having smashed furniture, mirrors, or whatever.

Who are the people who are always crying the blues? Who do you know who reeks of self-pity? Who keeps getting beat up for no reason at all? Whose eyes are bleary and bloodshot? It's those who spend the night with a bottle, for whom drinking is serious business. Don't judge wine by its label, or its bouquet, or its full-bodied flavor. Judge it rather by the hangover it leaves you with – the splitting headache, the queasy stomach. — Proverbs 23:19-33, *The Message* copyrighted ©

by Eugene H. Peterson, Used by permission of
NavPress Publishing Group.

What Shakespeare Knew

A splitting headache and queasy stomach are signs of a
hangover. But alcohol also kills brain cells and is a depressant.

*O God, that men should put an enemy in their
mouths to steal away their brains that we should,
with joy, pleasance, revel, and applause,
transform ourselves into beasts!* — William
Shakespeare, *Othello*

For those who believe beer is good for you, at least one
scientific study (LiveSci 2010) has linked beer drinking with
certain skin diseases, including psoriasis. Many beer drinkers
also become diabetics, as some of my cousins will testify.

So here's another Biblical statute that doubles as both a
moral principle and a health precept. Solomon warns us that
alcoholic drinks can "bite like a serpent." (Proverbs 23:29-35)

A Shot of Brain-Killer, Please

Some people believe "a little drink won't hurt,"
completely ignoring the evidence that alcohol kills brain cells and
that people who like to handle snakes have sometimes paid the
ultimate price. And I understand that, for those who have
experienced it, alcoholism can be a living hell.

Prohibiting wine and strong drinks might be seen as a moral law for priests in the temple, but it's also a precept for guarding our mental faculties so we can make wise decisions. This was shown in the case of the two Old Testament priests who weren't thinking straight when Yahweh sent fire down to destroy them for disobeying. Frank, too, as he ministered to his colleagues in that army dispensary, realized that following Solomon's proverbs actually makes our lives happier and healthier.

Liver Invasion

Laboratory tests show that alcohol can be blamed for liver problems in many heavy drinkers (Goldschmidt 2011). That's because our bodies interpret "the presence of alcohol as an invader," and call upon the liver to quickly neutralize this foreign substance. The damage to the liver, from this heavy toll "explains why alcoholics often end up suffering irreversible liver damage."

Among the cases of liver cirrhosis in the United States, only one in three has been shown to be caused by Hepatitis B or C (HerbalProvider.com 2009). The other two are a result of "high levels of alcohol consumption." Alcohol can also affect our mental and emotional well-being.

Once addicted to alcohol, we put ourselves at risk of developing "cardiovascular disease, malabsorption, chronic pancreatitis, alcoholic liver disease and cancer," as well as

172

damage to both the central and the peripheral nervous systems (Right-health2 2010).

If memory fails and confusion sets in, the poor addict may have developed either Wemicke-Korsakof Syndrome (Xiam 2009) or alcohol-induced psychosis, which has symptoms similar to schizophrenia. Although Vitamin B-1 may alleviate some symptoms of these two diseases, liver and pancreatic damage are seldom reversed (Larson 2010). And dead brain cells don't usually grow back, either.

While alcohol directly kills only the drinker's brain cells, it has also indirectly caused the deaths of many non-drinkers on the highways.

But cigarette smoke is deadly, too. New evidence keeps cropping up.

17. Where There's Smoke . . .

Know ye not that ye are the temple of God, and that the Spirit of God dwelleth in you? If any man defile the temple of God, him shall God destroy; for the temple of God is holy, which temple ye are.
— First Corinthians 3:16-17

When Frank returned from overseas duty, he attended college in the daytime and worked nights as a hospital orderly. Between rounds, one of the young doctors would often pass the time with Frank. This doctor, knowing Frank had been a medic in the Army, often discussed some of his cases with Frank.

"See that patient in there?" he pointed across the hall. "I had to amputate because there was a constriction in his leg, and it was going to turn gangrenous."

"How sad," Frank responded. "What do you think caused it?"

"Smoking," said the doctor, who snuffed out his own cigarette as he picked up his charts and prepared to go back to work. This was in the sixties, before smoking was banned in hospitals.

Frank was amazed that the doctor made no connection between his smoking and the possible harm it might do to his own body. But, having "been there and done that" myself, I realize that many of us have blind spots in our characters. For instance, even though I knew when I took up smoking that it shortens your wind, it never occurred to me, after several years of the habit, that smoking was the reason I couldn't keep up with the younger dancers. It was only after I quit smoking and got my wind back that I connected the effect to its cause.

In addition to ignoring published warnings because we enjoy a certain habit, most of us believe health laws are only for the *other* fellow. We often don't believe the consequences will affect US – until they do.

Smoke Gets in Your Eyes

Not only does smoke — like alcohol — kill brain cells, but it also leaves coal deposits on our lungs, turning them black and putting us at a higher risk for lung cancer, emphysema, and COPD (chronic obstructive pulmonary disease). The National Heart, Blood, and Lung Institute (NHBLI) estimates that more than 24 million Americans have COPD.

We put carbon monoxide detectors in our homes, so we won't become victims of carbon monoxide poison, but we often fill our homes with tobacco smoke, which does the same thing as carbon monoxide, only at a much slower rate. We rationalize that smoking helps us relax while we're slowly killing brain cells and turning our lungs black.

176

If you never thought smoke was deadly, remember that many people caught in out-of-control fires often die from smoke inhalation even though the flames never reach their bodies.

Sad, But True

When Frank and I were first married, we rented an apartment in a farmhouse for a few months. We lived upstairs over our very sociable landlords, the Chubbs.

From my bed I would often hear Mr. Chubb downstairs, coughing in the middle of the night.

"I had given up smoking," he confided one day, "but then a woman who smoked rented the upstairs apartment, and I started again. I wish you'd moved in then, instead of her," he told me. "Then I wouldn't have taken up this filthy habit again."

I've heard from several other ex-smokers that, if you go back to smoking after having once successfully quit, the habit is much harder to break the second time. And that seems to have been Mr. Chubb's problem. Entrapped a second time, he found the chains of addiction too hard to break. We heard that he died of lung cancer about a year after we moved out.

But lung cancer isn't the only ailment smoking can cause. Beryl, a close friend, blames BOTH her breast- and lung- cancers AND her COPD on the cigarettes she smoked for years. Mauve (mentioned earlier) and her husband both smoked for years. Mauve quit smoking when she was diagnosed with cancer, but he didn't. He developed emphysema while she was battling the first stages of her cancer. He huffed and puffed his way around the golf course, dangling a cigarette from his lips in his younger days and riding in a golf cart after he began having trouble breathing. A heavy drinker, he died six months after Mauve — of liver failure and pneumonia.

A Wrinkle in Time

It's common knowledge that women who smoke develop "crow's feet," those facial wrinkles in the corner of the eyes, sooner than women who don't smoke. And people addicted to smoking are "more likely [than nonsmokers] to face respiratory infections and several minor complaints such as coughs and colds" each year (Buzzle 2010).

Side Effects of Smoking:

Smoking also does the following: (1) stains teeth and gums, causes bad breath, and can lead to swollen gums and loose teeth; (2) often leads to infertility and increased asthma attacks; (3) lowers the birth weight of smoking mothers' babies; (4) contributes to macular degeneration and a higher rate of cataracts than among the general population; and (5) has been implicated in diabetic retinopathy, multiple sclerosis, Crohn's disease, and sudden infant death syndrome (Buzzle 2010).

In addition, several studies show that smoking "increases the risk for developing Type II Diabetes," and people with diabetes who smoke are "more likely to die prematurely from heart disease and stroke" than are diabetics who *don't* smoke (NIH 2010).

Last Minute Update

The National Cancer Institute recently funded a study of the effects of cigarette smoking on the human body and found disturbing results (Yahoo! 2011). They have issued a stark warning that genetic damage linked to cancer occurs so quickly that one of the toxins, called *phenanthrene*, "trashes DNA" within minutes of the first puff. The damage was "noticeable within 15 to 30 minutes after the volunteers finished their cigarettes and was found to create carcinogens in the blood and mutations in the cell's DNA."

I'm so glad I quit fifty years ago! Although I never got back my high soprano voice, my wind and endurance have returned – along with a strong sense of smell, for which I feel extremely blessed.

One of my friend's sisters smoked most of her life, stopping only during her pregnancies. She developed emphysema and was finally able to conquer the habit in her sixties, about ten years ago. She feels better physically, and her breathing has improved so much that she doesn't need to carry oxygen around with her any more during the daytime. She still needs it for sleeping, though.

An estimated 24 million Americans have COPD. If you're one of those unfortunate people, you might be interested to know that some researchers have found a way to help you breathe easier. A case-controlled study in Japan (RR 2009) found that "increasing soy consumption was associated with a decreased risk of COPD and breathlessness." Maybe in Japan they eat the green beans, grown organically, and make their own soy milk and tofu without additives.

The Last Word

At the very least, cigarette breath is unpleasant. And some longtime smokers eventually require leg amputation as a result of impaired blood flow. I don't know about you, but I wouldn't want to be confined to a wheel chair or have to drag an oxygen tank everywhere I go. I want to enjoy good health as I age. And speaking of growing old . . .

18. Moovin' and Groovin'

Go to the ant, thou sluggard; consider her ways, and be wise. — Proverbs 6:6

This proverb, by King Solomon, isn't just about being lazy and not saving up for the future. It's also a health principle, because the old adage, "Use it or lose it," is extremely relevant.

Have you ever noticed that the majority of older people in nursing homes are not there because they have a serious illness? They're there because they're too weak to make care of themselves! By age 65, one in four Americans cannot bathe, dress, eat, or get out of bed without help. And by age 85, the number has increased to fifty percent!

Why? Because the majority of us stop exercising after we marry and settle down to raise a family. When we stop using them, our muscles shrink.

Anyone who's ever broken an arm or a leg knows how stiff that arm or leg was when the doctor finally removed the cast. It takes a while to get the strength back in that limb. Why?

Because the principle, "Use it or lose it" is at work in all parts of our bodies.

In the forties and fifties, we children spent much of our free time outdoors playing games that required using our arm and leg muscles: hop scotch, jump rope, hide-and-seek, jacks, King of the Mountain, and group sports with balls or bean bags. In the summer, we roller-skated on the sidewalks. In winter, we dug out our sleds and ice skates and spent hours sliding down hills or skimming over the ice-covered ponds.

But in today's culture, with television and computers in every home, children spend less time exercising and more time sitting and munching. That explains much of the obesity among young people. But these youngsters are also losing muscle tone when they sit still all day.

We adults aren't doing much better. When America was a more rural society, our families grew much of our own food. All that hoeing-and-weeding was good for our waistlines and kept us physically strong. But, these days, most of us get our garden produce from a grocery store!

By age thirty-five, sedentary women are losing half a pound of muscle each year. And by age sixty-five the non-exercising woman has lost 40 percent of the muscle mass in her arms.

How do we keep from landing in a rest home where someone else has to bathe and dress us and help us out of bed in the morning? Walking is one answer. Walking helps with weight problems, too, and burns off fat quicker than running does.

While walking, we burn equal parts fat and sugar; but while running, we burn 80 percent sugar and only 20 percent fat.

If we Americans walked more and sat around less, even without a strenuous exercise program, our leg muscles would keep us mobile longer.

How to Stay Strong

Physiologists put a group of women in their 90's on a daily routine that included walking and leg exercises. In only eight weeks, the women in the program had tripled their leg strength. So apparently it's never too late to begin building up leg muscles.

The wisest way to begin an exercise program, if we've been sedentary for years, is to start walking, slowly increasing the time and distance as we're able. Walking is one of the least expensive forms of exercise, too, since there's no equipment to buy or classes we must take to become proficient at it. And while we're walking, we're exercising our legs *and* our heart muscle.

Being able to take care of ourselves when we reach our 80s and 90s is only one benefit of walking. A daily walking program also helps build resistance to disease by strengthening the lungs and heart muscle. Walking clears our head, keeps the blood flowing to the brain, and helps keep our memories sharp. People who suffer from insomnia usually sleep better, too, once they begin walking regularly.

The Big Four conditions brought on by an unhealthy lifestyle – heart disease, stroke, hypertension, and diabetes – all respond favorably to a walking program. As stated earlier, more than one doctor believes that half the people diagnosed as pre-diabetic will never actually succumb to diabetes if they begin exercising regularly.

Several researchers have also claimed that an exercise program will prevent osteoporosis, early dementia, and cancer, as well as the Big Four.

Getting Rid of Flab

Once we're well into a walking program, we should increase our speed and distance as we become more proficient, to get the most benefit. But we should never push ourselves so hard that we're breathing too hard to talk in phrases while we're exercising.

Many of us fear getting osteoporosis, and walking regularly can cut our risk of hip fracture by 40 percent. But NOT the risk of wrist fracture. And walking doesn't do a thing for arm flab, either.

Speaking of flab, parts of the body that aren't used frequently tend to accumulate "lazy" fat. The abdomen is the most notorious center of fat accumulation because we use those muscles the least. The second noticeable place is where the "love handles" form.

The only way to get rid of arm flab is to do strength training. But going to the gym isn't the only way to build arm strength. Many household chores will do wonders for our arm muscles and can help with deep breathing, too. When we sit at a desk or in front of a television set for long periods, we tend to "shallow" breathe, rather than breathing deeply.

Mopping, scrubbing, sweeping, ironing, vacuuming, and carrying groceries all require deep breathing and help keep our muscles active. Outside chores like yard-raking, lawn-mowing, washing and waxing the car, and shoveling snow will do the same thing.

Save Your Money and Your Strength!

Do you pay someone else to clean house for you? If so, your house-maids are building arm and muscle strength at your expense! In a group of sixty-year-old women who were tested, one-third of them couldn't even lift ten pounds! At that rate, if they don't begin strength training, they'll soon be one of those nursing-home residents that I mentioned earlier, who can't get out of bed alone and dress by themselves!

I greatly admired a military veteran who came into American Family Fitness® center while Frank and I were doing our water-robics early in the morning. This man would take off his artificial leg, lay it aside, and lower himself into the lap pool where he swam several laps. When he finished swimming, he lifted himself up over the side of the pool, using the arm muscles he'd developed since he lost his leg. He kept a pair of crutches nearby, but used them only in emergencies. This man was determined to take care of himself and not end up in a nursing home or be a burden on his family.

Hasten Recovery Time

Recovering from an injury? The staff in one hospital studied patients' recovery time and discovered that those who watched other people doing physical exercise recovered at a faster rate than those who didn't. It's possible that those patients exercised vicariously along with the physical exercisers, in their imagination, and sent positive health-building messages to their muscles and blood cells.

Brain Power

Physical exercise is one of the best activities we can do to regulate our metabolism and keep our minds sharp. To be adequately nourished, our brain cells require glucose and oxygen. Our blood supplies the needed glucose to our brains by itself, but we have a part to play in getting enough oxygen.

What are you doing to keep your brain cells well oxygenized? Take the simple test that follows, and check your oxygen quotient:

1. I follow a daily exercise regime   _____

2. I enjoy soap operas regularly   _____

3. I sing only at church   _____

4. Coffee keeps me awake at meetings   _____

5. My job requires hours at the computer   _____

(1) If you exercise regularly, you're probably getting all the oxygen you need as long as you're not hunched over a desk much of the day.

(2) Soap operas and suspenseful television programs do nothing to help us breathe deeply. Watching comedies that evoke a lot of laughter gets our diaphragms moving and forces us to breathe more deeply. Such actions allow us to take in more oxygen.

(3) If you're not a Caruso or a Liza Minnelli, sing in the shower where no one can hear you. Singing is one of the greatest exercises for the lungs, diaphragm, and vocal cords. It requires taking deep breaths, whereas humming doesn't.

(4) Whenever I must attend a meeting in a closed room, or even attend church services where the air doesn't circulate well and makes people drowsy, I carry a bottle of water with me. The water contains oxygen, which soda pop and caffeine drinks don't, and helps me cope with the lack of fresh air in the room. As shown earlier, soda and coffee actually pull water from our tissues. But drinking water helps me stay awake during the meeting, while getting some needed oxygen into my brain, and keeps me hydrated at the same time.

(5) We tend to slouch if we're at the computer for long periods. This causes shallow breathing. If we practice taking deep breaths whenever we take a bathroom break or answer the phone, we'll exercise our diaphragms and increase our oxygen supply.

Walk Your Way to Better Health

According to "Resources for Science Learning," walking improves our learning ability, concentration, and abstract reasoning. Older volunteers in a nursing home were put on a walking program. Those who participated showed an improved memory over those who didn't walk. These resources (Franklin 2011) also claim that "walking 20 minutes a day cuts our risk of having a stroke by 57 percent."

The saying, "Use it or lose it," goes for our brain cells, too. You may be surprised at the simple ways we can exercise our brains.

19. "B" is for Brain

I will praise thee; for I am fearfully and wonderfully made. — Psalm 139:14

Is growing senile a normal part of the aging process? Mara's husband thought so.

During lunch break one day I was showing the other teachers the puzzles and word games I played with my students on the first day of each semester, so they wouldn't think English classes had to be boring.

"Oh, my husband won't do any kind of exercise that requires thinking," Mara said.

"Why not?" the other teachers asked.

"He thinks we're given only so much brain-power, and he doesn't want to use his all up before he gets old."

It's true that brain cells get old and die off. But the research shows that the "use-it-or-lose-it" rule also goes for brain cells and cognitive function. In fact, they've found that it's the connectors – called synapses – between cells that keep our brains active, and not the cells themselves.

The more we use our brains, the better they perform for us. We've been told that most of us use only a tenth of our brain power. That's not true for everyone, though. Anyone who can do two things at once – like reading music while playing an instrument, or harmonizing a melody and keeping time with the beat, or repeating songs while jumping rope – is using more than a tenth of her brain.

And that's at least one reason why some older people stay alert while their same-age acquaintances show signs of dementia. We challenge our brains while we attend school, work at a career, or run a household; but when we no longer feel a need to find solutions, we stop using certain areas of the brain. In fact, our brains actually begin to shrink if we don't continue to challenge ourselves.

Pea Brains

Researchers measured the brains of animals caught in the wild just before they were sent to a zoo and then went back, a year or so later, and discovered that – having no need to hunt down game, protect a family, or find places to hide – the brains of those animals had shrunk while in captivity. With nothing to challenge them, these animals simply pace back and forth in their cages or fields, waiting for the zoo-keeper to bring their next meal.

A study of older people in retirement centers showed that those who put together jig-saw puzzles retain their spatial abilities longer than those who just watch television. Also, those who play bridge are noticeably more mentally alert than those who play only bingo. In addition, those who read only the comics in the Sunday newspaper are more apt to develop dementia than those who enjoy working crossword puzzles.

Volunteering their services to help others is one way many people keep their brains active. Others develop new hobbies when they reach retirement. One of the best ways people keep their minds sharp is to continually challenge themselves by learning new skills.

A Canadian study (Bowdler 2010) found that those people who grow up speaking more than one language are "less likely to develop forms of dementia, including Alzheimer's." That's probably because when people grow up in a home where two languages are spoken, they need to focus intently on the one being spoken at the time. This attention to detail strengthens their synapses and may be the reason their minds are more active through the years.

Win by Losing

One thing that can impair our reasoning ability, long-term memory, and coordination is being overweight. Resources at *Human Brain Mapping* showed that overweight people have four percent less brain tissue than people of normal weight. And obese people have eight percent less!

"Furthermore, the brains of overweight people looked eight years older than those of people of normal weight, and the brains of obese people looked a whopping sixteen years older!"

According to Dr. Paul Thompson, a UCLA professor, these results show "severe" brain degeneration (Raji 2009) and put people at a "much greater risk of Alzheimer's and other diseases that attack the brain."

If we have trouble understanding people who talk fast, we should do everything possible to lose any excess pounds we may be carrying around. Doing so may help us win back some cognitive functions we've lost.

Slow Down Your Aging!

Although it's been shown (BMJ 1996) that vegetarians have "lower mortality rates from several chronic degenerative diseases than do non-vegetarians," other factors are at work as well. Many who work with senior citizens suggest that exercise and a keen interest in life are essential for avoiding the diseases commonly associated with old age. The synapses between nerve cells grow stronger by performing new and challenging activities.

A Vitamin B-12 deficiency has been blamed for some cases of dementia, and most Alzheimer's patients have been found to have an excess of aluminum in their brains. But Dr. Sang Lee (2001) discovered that many people with heavy amounts of aluminum in their brains don't always get the disease. And although there are some studies linking Parkinson's disease to dairy products as well as to MSG, excitotoxins, and other harmful substances found in food additives, Dr. Lee believes our brains really begin aging when we stop making demands on them.

This famous Korean physician affectionately called the "Endorphin Doctor," teaches that disease always has a spiritual aspect as well (Lee 2001). Many aspects of our health depend on our attitude, as the following Bible verse states:

For as he thinketh in his heart, so is he.
— Proverbs 23:7, first part

Dr. Lee reports on some medical studies that prove his point. When a younger lion wins the battle over the male who was formerly the head of the pride, researchers discovered that the older, defeated lion's level of testosterone drops, even if he wasn't badly injured in the fight. Mentally, he knows he's been beaten and replaced by the new leader, so his system stops producing the abundant hormones needed as king of the pride (Lee 2001). The dominant males always produce more testosterone.

Another study was undertaken because certain nuns were developing Alzheimer's at a young age while others in the same nunnery remained mentally alert into their later years. Because they couldn't find any variance in the lifestyles of these nuns, the researchers asked for, and were given, permission to read the diaries of these nuns. The diaries of the healthy nuns contained many entries, with lots of writing in each, while the diaries of the ill nuns had hardly any entries at all. The researchers concluded that those who thought their lives had meaning and purpose felt they were making a worthwhile contribution to the community.

The other nuns, in the few entries they <u>did</u> make, appeared frustrated because they felt their lives were meaningless.

Lee believes that our brain sends messages to our various body parts, indicating that we no longer need them; and, as a result, organs and systems begin shutting down. If that's true then Proverbs 23:7 (back one page) holds true both physically and mentally, as shown in the following studies also recorded by Dr. Lee.

Expectations

Women who believe that "hot flashes" are a normal part of menopause — because their mothers had them — are more apt to experience them than women who have no such expectations. And here's another of Lee's observations: In cultures where child-bearing is emphasized as the woman's main reason for existence, many women who reach menopause believe they've served their purpose in life and are no longer worth much. It's then that their estrogen levels begin to drop, resulting in depression, insomnia, and hot flashes.

Some of Lee's colleagues studied the work habits of 100 owners and managers in Korean orphanages, of whom thirty had post-menopausal symptoms, while the other seventy didn't. The observers noticed that the ones with no symptoms hugged and touched the children on a daily basis, sharing their little concerns. The thirty with physical problems, on the other hand, showed no interest in the children and acted as if their work was "just a job."

Apparently, they felt their work was meaningless, and their brains were telling their bodies to stop producing estrogen.

As the Bible indicates, we're made up of body (physical), soul (mind), and spirit (the life force). We need all three to function at optimal levels; and Dr. Lee isn't the only physician who believes that all three can contribute to our health or our death (in the case of dying by degrees — as when a person has no reason to live and resigns herself to dying).

But that doesn't mean that our lifestyle doesn't affect our overall health, as we've seen with diabetes and sexually-transmitted diseases. Some studies (Greenwood 2011) show that "diets high in saturated fats can actually speed up the aging process in the brain." In addition, some health practitioners are classing Alzheimer's disease as *Type III Diabetes* because excess fat in the brain prohibits the glucose and insulin, required for healthy brain function, from entering the brain cells.

Protect Your Frontal Lobe

Several harmful agents can directly affect our brains, especially the frontal lobe, where our most important decisions are made. It's interesting that the top five are highly addictive:

1. Alcohol and other mind-altering drugs

2. Caffeine and nicotine

3. Flesh foods — especially salted, smoked, pickled, and preserved

4. Music with a hypnotic beat, especially the anapestic beat of rock music

5. Cheese, especially the aged kind: It contains "tyramine," which has been strongly implicated in migraine and cluster headaches (IGS 2011).

Since the frontal lobe is also the part of the brain where Yahweh communes with us, many see the use of alcohol and tobacco as "sins," rather than being unhealthy practices. But whether we view them as sins or as destructors of physical health and happiness, the research shows that taking up these habits can lead to bodily afflictions of various sorts.

Ten Steps to Building Brain Power

On the other hand, here are ten activities guaranteed to preserve brain cells and keep our minds alert and functional in our later years:

1. Work on brain teasers, including putting together jigsaw puzzles
2. Commit something to memory every week – such as Bible texts or great poetry
3. Find things to laugh about
4. Sing or play a musical instrument at least once a week
5. Listen to classical music

6. Get seven to eight hours of sleep each night
7. Exercise regularly; and if unable to exercise, practice deep breathing
8. Work on a project or a hobby that involves some type of physical exercise
9. Chew food thoroughly and eat a plant-based, nourishing diet including plenty of greens
10. Drink only water, preferably between meals

Taking care of our brain is only *one* aspect of living a healthy, productive life as we grow older. What about being sad? Can *that* shorten our lives?

20. Broken Spirits

A merry heart doeth good like a medicine, but a broken spirit drieth the bones. — Proverbs 17:22

Whenever I read the above text, it reminds me of our neighbors Edna and Bert. Because she was made Executrix of her mother-in-law's will, Edna divided the inheritance the way she thought was fair. One son had borrowed money from his parents and hadn't yet repaid it, so when Edna meted out the portions to each of the sons, she deducted the amount that son owed, which resulted in his receiving a smaller portion than she gave the others.

The angry son turned all his siblings against her and, to their dying day, none of Bert's relatives would speak to Bert or her. This really upset Edna, who developed all kinds of illnesses. Besides having a skin condition, she developed arthritis in her spine, diverticulitis, migraine headaches, and, finally, colon cancer.

Bert and Edna's diet wasn't the most healthful, but they weren't very big eaters; and I attribute most of her illnesses to a mental "pining away." Her bathroom shelf had so many medications on it that, whenever we visited, she had to move them all out of our children's reach.

I'm surprised her heart didn't fail her. Bert gave up cigar smoking before age fifty and lost weight when the doctor ordered him to. But neither he nor Edna cared much for physical exercise. Bert suffered mental anguish, both for loss of family relationships and for the way his relatives treated Edna. He and Edna hardly ever smiled, went walking, or played music to make them forget their troubles. It didn't help that all Bert's relatives lived close by, and they couldn't help but bump into them and endure their icy rejection in grocery stores or at community events.

After her first bout with colon cancer, Edna was caught between a rock and a hard place when she took a secretarial job at her church. The Board of Deacons didn't always agree with the new minister's decisions. When the deacons would chastise Edna for making changes in the church bulletin, she'd learn that it was really the new minister who'd made the change. And when the minister gave her orders, the deacons would make changes that would result in the minister's verbally attacking Edna. She finally quit that job, which had been her only source of self-fulfillment after Bert's relatives stopped talking to them.

When Edna's cancer returned, Bert started having hallucinations and ended in the same hospital with her – but on a different floor. When he had to be placed in a nursing home where someone could keep an eye on him, it was too much for Edna. They died within weeks of each other, and the only relatives at their funerals were from Edna's side of the family. Although she and Bert didn't follow many rules of healthful living, I'm sure their sadness and grief were the major cause of their illnesses and early deaths. Edna died before all of her older siblings.

An inspired Christian visionary (EGW 1982) wrote this: "Sadness deadens the circulation in the blood vessels and nerves, and also retards the action of the liver. It hinders the process of digestion and of nutrition, and has a tendency to dry up the marrow of the whole system." In Edna's case, the statement really rings true.

> *A sound heart is the life of the flesh. . .*— Proverbs 14:30, first part

> *. . . but by sorrow of the heart the spirit is broken.*
> — Proverbs 15:12, last part

We can equate grief with sadness because both emotions make us feel miserable. Both can cause regrets, either for something we've done or something we've neglected to do. And I've seen prolonged anguish causing a devastating effect on various people's health.

Dr. Sang Lee says our heart muscles can begin dying when we grieve (Lee 2001). His statement reminds me of Annette. Her case seems to be a classic example of Lee's teaching.

Annette was NOT a sparkly, effervescent person when I first met her. She had a sad, Mona Lisa-like smile. One day at a religious gathering, I asked if her husband was a Christian because I'd never seen him at any church functions.

"He used to be," she admitted. "But he stopped attending church, and I think it's my fault."

I didn't ask why, because I didn't really know her very well and didn't want to pry. She didn't drink water, either, and often complained of not being able to remember something after she'd read it. So she was probably somewhat dehydrated.

But I watched the next few years as she suffered through several cancer operations, and she never struck me as a person struggling to regain her health. Maybe she thought her bouts of cancer were "punishment" for whatever she thought she'd done to make her husband stop coming to church. All I know is that she wasn't a "happy camper." She seemed to me to be just waiting for death to come and claim her.

And Janelle's story is similar. After watching her husband suffer through years of cancer treatments, she was physically and mentally worn out. When, at a routine physical, she discovered she also had cancer, with only six months to live, she refused all treatments. She was going to die anyway, she thought, so why prolong her suffering with radiation and chemotherapy's devastating side effects?

By the way, except for growing extremely tired by nightfall, Janelle experienced hardly any pain until about three weeks before she died. She just kept losing weight until she finally pined away.

It's not unusual for some spouses to die within a few years of each other, especially if the one left behind doesn't move past the initial grief.

Howard

Dodee's husband died suddenly in his fifties and, after her children were grown, she went back to school to get a nursing degree. Eventually she became a Visiting Nurse and enjoyed making her rounds and getting to know her patients. One of her cancer patients was dying, and the husband was beside himself with grief.

One day, shortly after the man's wife had died, Dodee stopped by, to see how he was faring, and found him face down on the floor. Howard had devoted his life to his wife, and now he just wanted to die. Somehow, Dodee encouraged him to go on living.

Howard and Dodee started seeing each other and were married about six months later. They were married only a year when he had a gallbladder attack and was hospitalized. When the surgeon began to operate, though, he discovered Howard's body was riddled with cancer. This was back in the early seventies before CAT scans and MRI tests were common.

In his weakened condition, Howard never recovered from the surgery. He died in the hospital a couple days later.

The startling thing was that when Dodee went to find the insurance papers, in the place he'd told her they'd be, all Howard's affairs had been perfectly arranged in order, as if he knew he wouldn't be coming out of the hospital and was trying to make all the paperwork easy for her.

After the funeral Dodee declared that Howard's cancer was a direct result of grieving for his first wife. Dodee believed his heart had started dying when the wife died, and it wasn't strong enough to carry him through both gallbladder surgery and the recovery period – even if the cancer hadn't metastasized.

Live Long and Die Short

An old German proverb says, "We live too short and die too long," a statement that's certainly true if we begin abusing our health at a young age.

One way to stay healthy and young at heart is to laugh often. Children laugh as many as 400 times a day, and a few adults laugh as many as 75 times a day. But the majority of us laugh fewer than 25 times a day. Not only does laughter cause creativity in the brain, but it fills our lungs with oxygen which our brains, blood cells, and lungs all need to stay flexible and to function properly.

"People begin to die when they give up in any area of life," says Dr. Lee, even if all they do is to stop calling family members when they're lonely.

Unhappy people live too short and die too long. We should find a purpose for life, a healthy reason for existing, and a passion for living. Then maybe we'll start living longer and dying shorter.

Would you like to help someone live longer? Here's one secret:

Heaviness in the heart of man maketh it stoop, but a good word maketh it glad. — Proverbs 12:23

The world is full of hateful, mean-spirited people. But we can make the world a happier place and even lift people's spirits to the point of strengthening their immune system if we understand that the above Bible verse is one of life's health-giving secrets.

Building people up, praising their efforts, and finding something pleasant to say to them is sometimes the best medicine we can administer.

On the other hand, if we snap at people and criticize them, the Bible says we're piercing their hearts and may cause them to begin dying.

And what about forgiving people? The Bible says Yahweh will forgive us only if we first forgive others who've hurt us. That precept appears to be salvational, doesn't it? But let's look beyond that spiritual application and see how the act of forgiving relates to our health and wellness.

21. Cells That Remember

And forgive us our debts, as we forgive our debtors. — Matthew 6:13

Since this book is about health issues, let's read the above prayer as if it were a health principle, which it is, as well as a moral precept. As several medical studies show, we damage both mind and body when we harbor a grudge.

Brian Tracy says "most unhappiness and psychosomatic illness is caused by the inability to forgive," which often results in anxiety and depression (Tracy 1993). Dr. Bruce Lipton, formerly of Stanford Medical School, explains how negative feelings bring about illness. He says we may develop wrong beliefs, called "cellular memories" that lodge *not just in the brain* but also in cells all over the body. He further blames 95 percent of our disease and illnesses on the stress these negative beliefs, or cellular memories, place on the cells of our internal organs (Peck 2010).

Harvard Medical School blames stress for the many illnesses that make us sick and tired and drain us of energy. And Southwestern University Medical Center in Dallas Texas says much of our stress is from cellular memories that have never been healed (Peck 2010).

Some negative cellular memories, implanted in us by the time we reach age six, may develop into chronic stressors if we dwell on them through the years.

.

Effects of Stress on the Cellular Level

Chronic stress —
1) lies at the root of "burn out"
2) inhibits the body's natural *DNA repairing system* from fighting off cancer and other degenerative diseases
3) weakens the immune system
4) affects the body's ability to metabolize fat, leading to weight problems

Our friend Maribelle won't visit a certain institution because years ago someone there hurt her feelings. She says, "They're still there" – the ones who inflicted the hurt on her. Maribelle is usually pale, doesn't laugh very often, and – although a health-conscious vegetarian — recently suffered a stroke. It's possible her negative memories are keeping her cells in a constant state of stress.

These negative memories that lodge in cells all over our body are, I believe, one of the reasons so many people are consulting alternative healing modalities such as hypnotism, aromatherapy, massage therapy, energy healing, yoga, reflexology, and others. *Modern Medicine*, which merely treats the symptoms of disease, has not been able to alleviate people's stress-causing negative memories.

Dr. McMillan tells another story of an elderly patient's blood pressure, which usually hovered around 200.

One day her systolic was up to 230, but the doctor didn't want to alarm her. So he kept his voice casual as he remarked, "Your pressure's up today."

"It should be," she answered. "I just had a heated argument with another patient in your waiting room."

McMillan was surprised that such a cultured, intelligent woman would "blow up" at a stranger who apparently provoked her with his chatter. "She could have had a stroke right there in my office," he reported.

"Arguments and verbal duels cause *many*, and aggravate *all*, cases of high blood-pressure," he claims (McMillan 1967).

Letting Go

If your feelings have been hurt by somebody, "you have the choice of constantly reliving the pain or letting it go by forgiving the offender" (Azur 1997). Two researchers at the University of Northern Iowa studied a dozen incest survivors (Jiskha 2011) and discovered that "those who forgave their abusers had more hope and less anxiety and depression than those who didn't." A year later, a follow-up exam showed that those forgivers *remained* more hopeful and less depressed than the ones who refused to forgive.

Another study was done on abused people who wanted help with forgiving their perpetrators. One group simply forgave from a distance, by letter or by journal-writing. The second group was given the assignment of going to their former abusers and doing something beneficial for them – such as mowing their lawn, or taking them shopping or to a doctor's appointment.

Afterward, the group that wrote out their forgiveness felt relieved, but they didn't show the same happiness and lightheartedness as the group that went a step further. The Bible calls this additional step "going the second mile" and "heaping coals of fire on your enemy." It's a health rule, folks, and aids in lifting our spirits and eliminating depression. Even those diagnosed with clinical depression can benefit from helping others.

Some people believe that forgiving someone else takes away their feeling of control. But this is simply a negative *false* belief. When we continually relive the painful episode in our minds, we're bombarding our cells with toxic messages and giving the other person power to continually hurt us. Once we forgive the perpetrator, most of us feel liberated and light-hearted, as if we've suddenly been relieved of an extremely heavy burden. Brian Tracy believes "forgiveness is a SELFISH act" (Tracy 1993) because it releases us from stress, ailments, and negativity — and leads to "happiness, peace of mind, and long life."

Someone sent me this quotation by Max Lucado that sums it up well: "Forgiveness is unlocking the door to set someone free and realizing you were the prisoner."

Family Rupture

When her daughter May died, Dee waited for May's husband Ken to repay the large sum of money he'd borrowed for May's hospital bills and medical treatment. When the insurance money came in, though, he went out and bought a Cadillac instead. Because he didn't offer to repay the loan, Dee felt Ken was ungrateful and changed her will. She decided to cut him out entirely and leave his and May's share to his three daughters.

About a year later Ken died, and his and May's three daughters got the Cadillac and their parents' two houses. Thinking it over, Dee decided Ken's daughters had already inherited more from their own parents than her two remaining daughters, Hillary and Opal, would get when she died. So she revised her will again, leaving Ken's daughters out completely.

When Dee died several years later, May's daughter Gina wouldn't go to her grandmother's memorial service because she learned she wouldn't be receiving any of the inheritance she'd expected. She even stopped communicating with her two aunts, Hillary and Opal.

That was fifteen years ago, and I figured everyone had made up by now. So on our last visit, I asked Hillary and Opal how Gina was doing.

"Oh, we don't hear from her any more. She's never forgiven us for executing the will according to Mom's wishes," Hillary told me.

"She must be okay," Opal added. "If anything happened to her, one of her daughters would let us know."

"Gina acts as if we don't exist," Hillary said, "But I'm not going to lose any sleep over it. Life's too short. I'm going to enjoy the little time I have left."

Hillary has the right attitude. Desiring good health and a cheerful attitude, she refuses to let a niece's aloofness bother her. As the famous Booker T. Washington once said, "I will not let any man [person] reduce my soul to the level of hatred."

I feel sorry for Gina, though, because they say she's obese and may suffer from colitis or irritable bowel syndrome. One doctor has said that 96 percent of his patients with mucous colitis admitted to resentment in their relationship issues. And ulcerative colitis, an even more serious condition, can be caused by emotional turmoil (McMillan 1967).

If reliving negative past events affects our bodies at the cellular level, could worry and extreme fear also affect our overall health? Let's look at some other research.

22. Worrisome Expectations

Take therefore no thought for the morrow: for the morrow shall take thought for the things of itself. Sufficient unto the day is the evil thereof.
— Matthew 6:34

Dr. McMillan tells the story of a patient whose hands were crippled with rheumatoid arthritis.

"Did you fall and injure them?" the doctor asked.

"No, there was a panther loose in our territory when I was nine years old. Every time I had to run through the woods to get home from school, I was petrified the panther would attack me. My hands have been crippled ever since."

This man realized his deformity was caused by that traumatic period in his childhood; but not everyone can trace the cause of his ailments so easily.

Fear and worry, often caused by financial and emotional distress, have been linked to anxiety, depression, insomnia, and migraines. Mental health authorities point to the home foreclosure crisis as contributing to the recent surge in stress and anxiety, resulting in an increase in suicides.

During the 2008 housing debacle psychologists reported that one of every four patients was suffering from some type of mental illness, including depression.

Besides causing arthritis, depression, and migraine headaches, prolonged worry can also result in glandular disturbances. Continual strain on the adrenal glands can result in infertility in females. And over-stimulation of the thyroid gland can result in fatigue, poor circulation, and weight problems.

Extreme Cases

Negative emotions can damage our bodies at least three ways:

1) The first way is through cellular memories, described in the previous chapter. We know a young woman addicted to pain medication. She tried to get rid of her addiction by going "cold turkey" but landed in the hospital following a panic attack. Someone offered to send her to a health institute where the staff could supervise her as she came off the medication, and she made the trip. But when she got there, she was so fearful of having another panic attack that she refused to follow the program. How sad, especially as the caretakers there were trained and equipped to treat those willing to take the necessary steps to rid themselves of that addiction.

Today, this woman complains of fuzzy thinking and chronic fatigue. She also has a heart problem, no doubt caused by the many medications she believes she needs.

2) The second is hypochondria. Everyone seems to have met at least one hypochondriac somewhere. Some, no doubt, are starved for affection and use their supposed ailment to get attention. However, a large number are driven by such fear (of cancer or other life-threatening diseases) that they actually make themselves sick.

My friend Rita told me about the fears of her mother whose father and older brother had both died of heart attacks, and she feared she would too. Every time she heard of someone having a heart attack, Rita's mother would have a panic attack with pains in her chest. She was sure she was having a heart attack herself until an EKG would show that her heart was fine. Even when her mother died, Rita said, it was from cancer and not from a heart attack.

Other hypochondriacs experience changes in appetite, weight gain, fatigue, and decreased interest in sex. Many even lose their zeal for living – worried that they have a fatal disease when their real problem might be anxiety or depression (Wikipedia 2010).

3) The third condition has been given a medical name: GAD, or generalized anxiety disorder. Anxiety disorders are among the most common mental illnesses (Worry 2011). About six percent of Americans will have GAD sometime in their life although twice as many women as men will develop the disorder.

GAD even has a web site devoted specifically to it (ADAA 2011). People with this disorder experience exaggerated worry and tension, anticipate disaster momentarily, and don't know how to break the worry cycle. Although some authorities blame the condition on a chemical imbalance in the brain – which can be caused by poor diet and lifestyle, we know that negative thinking can also produce changes in brain cells. And so can dehydration, as noted earlier.

Nervous Blood Clotting

In 1951 Dr. David Macht measured the number of minutes required for the blood of fifty normal persons to clot, and he "compared [those figures] with the clotting time of the blood of a hundred nervous" persons. Here's what he discovered:

Patients	Clotting time
50 normally happy people	8-12 minutes
50 apprehensive people	4-5 minutes
50 highly nervous people	1-2 minutes

The doctor was surprised to discover that people's nervous state could influence their blood's clotting tendency *to such a great degree* (McMillan 1967). We can see — from his observations — why extreme worry or anxiety may bring on a heart attack or stroke without much warning.

Some people are more apt to worry than others, but notice the following statistics:

- 40 percent of what we worry about will never happen,
- 30 percent of what we fear or worry about are related to things that happened in the past and can't be changed,
- 10 percent of our worries are considered by most to be insignificant issues,
- 12 percent of things we worry about are health issues that will not occur.
- This means that 92 percent of the things we fear or worry about will never take place. (Fear 2011)

Let's receive the Savior's admonition, "Take no thought for the morrow," as an additional health prescription so we don't *worry ourselves sick!*

Whatever our problems, we can do as the song says and "take it to the Lord in prayer."

Some doctors have begun to study the power of prayer on their patients. What they've discovered is amazing.

217

23. Prayer Power

The effectual fervent prayer of a righteous man availeth much. — James 5:16, last part

*R*eader's Digest reported on a nationwide study of 21,000 people, showing that those who prayed and attended religious services more than once a week had a seven-year longer life expectancy than those who never attended services (AF 2009). In fact, traditional religious beliefs benefit our health, says Duke University professor Harold Koenig, M.D. (2010). He says people who pray tend to get sick less often and suffer depression less often. When they do become depressed, he claims they recover more quickly than people who don't pray.

Koenig also quotes results of several studies at Dartmouth and Yale, as well as those at Duke University:

- Hospitalized people who never attended church had an average stay of three times longer than people who attended regularly.
- Heart patients were 14 times more likely to die following surgery if they did not participate in a religion.

- Elderly people who never or rarely attended church had a stroke rate double that of people who attended regularly.
- In Israel, religious people had a forty percent lower death rate from cardiovascular disease and cancer.

(Koenig 2010)

Although participating in organized religion can promote healthy living by discouraging such behaviors as smoking, alcohol, drug use, and promiscuity through social pressure, there's evidence that prayer alone can play a contributing factor in disease recovery.

Don't Confuse Me with the Facts!

Although humanists and evolutionists frown upon the mixture of religion and medicine, note this:

> In a controversial study carried out by cardiologist Randolph Byrd (*Southern Medical Journal*, July 1988), nearly 400 heart patients were randomly assigned to either a group that was prayed for by a home prayer group or a control group. This was a methodologically rigorous double-blind study designed to eliminate the psychological placebo effect. In such a study, neither the patient nor doctor knows who is receiving the intervention (i.e., prayer). Patients who received prayer had better health outcomes, including a reduced need for antibiotics and a lower incidence of pulmonary edema (Johnston 2010).

In his report, Johnston also quotes the work of John Stucki, a prayer researcher who carried out "double-blind studies evaluating the effects of distant prayer on the body's electromagnetic fields." In Stucki's Colorado Springs laboratory they measured the electrical activity in both the brain and body surface of the patients. The groups who prayed were nearly 1000 miles away in California, yet the results showed that the electrical activity in the people prayed for was "significantly altered compared to controls" (Johnston 2010).

Pray Along Life's Pathway

David Larson, MD, MSPH, and president of the National Institute for Healthcare Research, says research on the power of prayer in healing has nearly doubled in the past ten years. According to him, "Even the NIH – which refused to even review a study with the word *prayer* in it four years ago – is now funding one prayer study (webmd 2011) through its Frontier Medicine Initiative." This study, with Johns Hopkins University School of Medicine if I'm correct, will include women who have early-stage breast cancer. Only half of the women will know that people in their religious group will be praying for them. If I had breast cancer, I'd want to be in the group being prayed for!

When Frank came home from the hospital after his heart attack, with doctor's orders not to get angry, he knew he had a problem. He'd gotten angry so often that it had become a habit to blow up whenever he was hungry, tired, or upset. Worried that his next bout of anger would kill him, he began praying for supernatural help. He knew he couldn't break that habit on his own. If you met him today, you'd know that his prayers have been answered. It's thirty years since his heart attack; he's still alive, and he hardly ever blows up!

Praying for Our Enemies

Some psychologists are starting to agree with the Bible's admonition when it says to "pray for your enemies." They've found that prayer, as a coping mechanism, helps people calm down and view the world with less aggressiveness.

Psychology professor Brad Bushman at Ohio State University reports on three separate studies relating the effects of prayer on anger. Although atheists didn't participate, the person's religious affiliation had no bearing on the results. People who prayed –

- Were better able to deal with negative emotions
- Reported lower levels of anger at the person than those who simply thought about the other person
- Tended to get less angry about the turn of events and blame the situation, as compared to those who didn't pray at all and tended to blame other people rather than the event.

The above research was reported online at Believe (2011), and contains a link to the studies themselves.

Grace and Gratitude

Occasionally I've prayed aloud for people, with their permission, when they were upset. Nearly all of them afterward said, "I feel better now." So even hearing someone pray for you apparently eases stress.

Some researchers even claim that saying grace before meals "settles your heart and mind and prepares you to eat with a positive spirit — a real digestive aid!" At the very least, it forces you to calm down, if you're upset about something, before you begin eating — giving your digestive juices a few moments to relax (Psych 2010). In fact, "scientists have found that eating in a relaxed state may be even more healthful than chewing one's food thoroughly."

Stress has been shown to cause digestive problems, disrupting the "gut flora and contributing to the development of food allergies," and psychologists have noted that people's "ability to experience and express gratitude is a key to . . . overall health" (Psych 2010).

More and more doctors are admitting that Christians who pray a lot, and strongly believe that Yahweh intervenes in their lives, suffer fewer stress-related ailments!

They're making new discoveries about sleep too, as we'll see in the next chapter.

223

24 Sleep, Sweet Sleep

The sleep of a laboring man is sweet, whether he eat little or much: but the abundance of the rich will not suffer him to sleep. — Ecclesiastes 5:12

According to the Bible text above, those who depend on their wealth, or worry about losing it, cannot enjoy the good night's sleep that the average working person enjoys. In addition, anxiety about future events can also cause us to lose sleep, even when we go to bed at a decent hour. We're told that as many as 60 million Americans suffer from insomnia. Some have trouble falling asleep and others can't stay asleep all night; some have the problem as many as three nights a week, and others are continually plagued with some type of insomnia.

Adequate sleep –
- Allows the body and mind to repair and rejuvenate themselves
- Slows down the aging process
- Boosts the immune system
- Helps with weight control

- Improves brain function, resulting in higher test scores in students

(7-Steps 2011)

In fact, sleeping well helps keep you alive longer. "Among humans, death from all causes is lowest among adults who get seven to eight hours of sleep nightly, and significantly higher among those who sleep less than seven or more than nine hours" (Lambert 2005). Yet we Americans sleep 1.5 hours, or 20 percent, less than our parents did.

Sleep Stages

According to research, we sleep in stages, and although we dream most during Stage Five, called Rapid Eye Movement or REM, we can also dream in stages three and four, although most people don't remember the dreams occurring in those stages.

In Stage One, we're just dropping off to sleep, and our muscles may twitch as our brain begins slowing down.

In Stage Two, our body temperature drops, and our breathing and heart rates slow down as we drift off into a deep sleep.

Our brains produce Delta waves in Stage Three, which is more common in children. Adults appear to spend less time in this stage.

Stage Four is the most restful stage. By now our muscles have relaxed into an almost-paralyzed state so that we don't act out our dreams.

In REM, or Stage Five, our brains show the most activity. Even our breathing and heart rates speed up. In this period, our dreams are most vivid as our eyes flutter; and these are the dreams we're most likely to remember when we're wakened suddenly.

Researchers claim we dream many times each night, because we go through these five stages several times – as many as five – in a single night. No matter what occurs during the final stage, studies show that lack of sleep effects long-term memory and causes a decrease in our productivity on the job.

Insomnia

There's nothing as frustrating as going to bed early, in order to be well rested for the next day's activities, only to toss and turn for hours while sleep eludes us. Many people turn to sleeping pills because they can't fall asleep naturally.

Apparently, I'm not the only one who's experienced this problem. According to the *Los Angeles Times*, one in ten Americans has trouble either falling asleep or staying asleep the whole night; and the number increases during times of financial crises (7/30/2011).

Although Dr. Duke's team found an average 70 side effects in the 5,600 drug labels they examined, and published their results in *Archives of Internal Medicine* (NHD 2011), over

40 percent of Americans still use sleeping pills, either regularly or occasionally.

Yet that *Los Angeles Times* article listed at least four dangers these people face:

- dependence
- next-day-drowsiness
- memory loss
- sleep-walking

And according to Dr. Kripke's studies, sleeping pills were "associated with significantly increased *mortality*" (that's *death*, folks). In his latest book he says those who take sleeping pills occasionally have an increased death rate of 10-15 percent, while those who take them nightly increase their death rate by 25 percent (Dark 2011).

Kripke found documented evidence of sleep problems in recovering alcoholics and also stated that about two-thirds of the sleeping pills sold in America are taken chronically for several years, increasing those users' risk for cancer.

The fact that so many sleeping pills are being prescribed and sold shows how prevalent the loss of sleep is becoming in our society.

Some doctors claim early evening sleep fills our memory banks, and the sleep we get before midnight is twice as beneficial as any sleep we get after that.

Although there's no empirical proof yet, it's thought that children's brains might use the sleep cycle to entrench events or language skills in their memory and that adult brains use the down-time to make sense of past events and mentally prepare themselves for the following day's projects. It's also thought that our brains use sleep time to transfer thoughts from short-term memory to our long-term memory.

Some people's arm and leg muscles remain active, even in the fifth stage; a departure from the norm. A few sleep disorders, like sleepwalking or lashing out as we dream, may be related to over-stimulation or acidity in the blood.

For instance, the mother of one of my dance pupils was horrified in the middle of the night to discover her daughter standing outside on the fire escape in her nightgown. The mother complained to the pediatrician who suggested that they cut out her daughter's baby vitamins since the girl was now ten years old. As soon as they eliminated the vitamins, the girl's sleepwalking ceased.

Physical Ailments Due to Sleep Deprivation

Without adequate sleep, our immune systems are weakened. The number of white blood cells decreases; and the activity of those remaining slows down. Our bodies also produce fewer growth hormones (Emed 2011), and our ability to metabolize sugar declines, turning it into body fat.

Lack of sleep may also be implicated in diabetes, immune-system dysfunctions, impaired job performance, and safety issues, such as medical errors (Lambert 2005) and car accidents. In America, 23 percent of us fall asleep at the wheel, causing 100,000 automobile accidents resulting in over 1500 fatalities each year (7-Steps 2011).

Even though we're warned to get eight hours of sleep each night, from 50 to 70 million Americans "live on the brink of mental and physical collapse due to lack of sleep" (7-Steps 2011). The National Institute of Health estimates the loss of productivity in the workplace caused by sleep-deprived people to be at least $50 billion each year.

A study of children from kindergarten through fourth grade found that ten percent of children fell asleep in class, an indication of poor sleeping habits and/or sleep disturbances. One cause of such disturbances was found to be connected to children's having television sets and/or computer games in their bedrooms. Yet another study linked sleep deprivation to a 420 percent increased risk of obesity in six-year-olds (Sleep 2008).

Death may be either a direct cause or a side effect of sleep deprivation. There's also a newly published study claiming women who work the night shift or sleep in lighted bedrooms suffer from breast cancer more than women who work days and sleep in darkened bedrooms.

Our bodies make melatonin while we sleep, and melatonin has been shown to repress the growth of tumors. Researchers claim that a drop in melatonin, from lack of sleep or sleeping in a well-lit room, sets the stage for liver cancer and malignant breast tumors (Dr. Kim 2011).

Some people pride themselves at being able to function on only a few hours' sleep each night. But another study found that people who sleep less than four hours per night are three times more likely to die within the next six years (Men's 2011).

Tips for the Weary

Note these excellent tips for falling asleep: (Adapted from 2004 *Bottom Line Year Book*)

1. Relax an hour before bedtime
2. After noon, avoid caffeine
3. Don't drink alcohol at night
4. Get up and go to bed at the same time every day
5. Exercise for a half hour, early in the day (not before bedtime)
6. Have a bedtime ritual that you perform every night
7. Do not listen to the news or any exciting television programs before going to bed
8. Listen to soft music or relaxation tapes after you get in bed
9. Don't keep computers or electronic devices in your bedroom

10. Keep the room dark at nighttime, and sleep with the window open at least a crack, to let in fresh air

Nightly muscle cramps can sometimes be relieved by drinking three glasses of water before returning to bed. Many practitioners believe these cramps are a symptom of mild dehydration and suggest drinking eight glasses of water every day to prevent recurrences.

Little children often dread bedtime because they don't want to stop what they're doing, but by the time we're adults we usually look forward to a good night's rest. The opposite is sometimes true of vacations. Children love picnics, trips to new places, and a fun day at the beach. But many adults are workaholics and find excuses for not taking vacations.

Vacations not only rest our bodies, from the everyday routine; but if we don't try to cram too much into them, they also relax the mind and refresh us spiritually. That may be why Yahweh built so many vacations into the Biblical calendar.

25. Time Off

There remaineth therefore a rest to the people of God. — Hebrews 4:9

According to the Apostle Paul, Yahweh's people are destined to enter some kind of rest that the Israelites of old didn't enter when they wandered forty years in the wilderness. You can read Paul's whole soliloquy in Hebrews Three and Four.

What is this rest that they didn't enter? The word *rest* in this verse comes from the Greek word "sabbatismos" (#4520 in *Strong's Concordance*), which comes from the Hebrew word "Shabbat," meaning *the seventh* — or *the weekly*— day of rest.

The Bible tells us that the Jewish nation, before their Babylonian captivity, *outwardly* celebrated the holy days Yahweh hallowed and blessed. But *inwardly*, they were just "showing up" at the synagogue on the Sabbaths and Yahweh's other mandated feasts. We get our first hint of this in Isaiah 1:13-15 when the prophet declares that Yahweh hated their offerings, their Sabbaths, and their new moons.

Why would Yahweh hate the holy days that He himself instituted, especially since He pronounced everything that He made "good"? We learn the real reason in Amos 8:5+6 where the prophet explains Yahweh's displeasure by telling us that, when they should have been enjoying the sacred hours, the people were saying to themselves: *"When will the new moon be gone, that we may sell corn? And the Sabbath, that we may set forth wheat, making the ephah small, and the shekel great, and falsifying the balances by deceit? That we may buy the poor for silver, and the needy for a pair of shoes; yea, and sell the refuse of the wheat?"*

In other words, they were not only losing the special rest and communion with Him that Yahweh wanted them to enjoy, but they were also breaking the heart of the commandment by using Yahweh's hallowed hours to devise ways to make more money, by cheating people and oppressing the poor. (See also Amos 5 and Ezekiel 22:8+26.)

By putting their greed and love of money first, they never realized the spiritual value or the health implications of true Sabbath-keeping. Yes, our body slows down when we sleep but, since our minds are still busy in Stages Four and Five, Yahweh knew our minds needed more rest than we can obtain in a few hours of sleep.

When we cease from toil on Yahweh's weekly Sabbath and remember all the blessings He has bestowed on us, we not only give our minds and bodies a rest from our everyday routine, but we also have the opportunity to refresh our spirits and exercise different parts of the brain from the ones we use during our daily chores. Varied activities strengthen the synapses between brain cells and keep us alert, especially if we spend some of the Sabbath hours helping others, singing songs of praise, visiting shut-ins, and memorizing Scripture or inspirational poetry.

We know that exercising six days a week is fine, but seven days of heavy physical exercise is too much for the average person. Seven consecutive days of heavy labor, of running a business, or of continual pressure to achieve a sales quota, also put stress on our immune systems.

I've been told by more than one person in the medical field that Sabbath-keepers' heart rates actually *drop* on the Sabbath. I was repeating this news to a male Sabbath-keeper who replied haughtily, "Well, I know for a fact that mine doesn't!"

When I looked at him in surprise, he responded, "I have a pace-maker."

So, naturally, there are exceptions.

However, the medical literature suggests that surgeons don't know if their organ-transplant recipients' bodies have fully accepted the new organ until either the seventh or fourteenth day after surgery. And dental surgeons usually want to check their patients seven days after an intrusive procedure, recognizing that the human body runs on a seven-day cycle.

Different Apps for Different Chaps

During World War II, Great Britain implemented a 74-hour work week, hoping to increase factory production. The people, however, couldn't keep up the pace (Ludington 1995).

After some experimentation, they found that a "48-hour work week, with regular breaks, plus one day of rest each week, resulted in maximum efficiency."

Germany also increased its work week during the war and tried keeping its factories running twenty-four hours a day. But machinery kept breaking down, and there was no time between shifts for it to be repaired. Also, great numbers of people were getting hurt on the job from lack of sleep.

The French, too, learned something interesting. As part of the French Revolution, the nation of France operated on a ten-days-per-week calendar for about 12 years, and implemented it again for 18 days in 1871; but during that time France was "out of synch" with the other nations.

> This unique calendar was finally abolished *"because having a ten-day working week gave workers less time to rest (only one day off every ten days instead of every seven); because the equinox was a mobile date to start every new year (a fantastic source of confusion for almost everybody); and because it was incompatible with the secular rhythms of trade fairs and agricultural markets"* (Wikipedia 2011).

In America's fast-paced society, people often feel pressured to overwork. Frank has told me, many times, that if it weren't for the Sabbath, he'd have died from overwork years ago. Some people tax themselves six days of the week and must catch up on their sleep on their one day off. And some self-employed people often work a seven-day week and rest only when their annual vacation rolls around.

But driving ourselves too hard can take a toll on our bodies, as one of our neighbors can testify. He was diagnosed with multiple sclerosis when he was only 28. Telling us about it, he said, "It's my own fault. I pushed too hard, keeping late hours and working two jobs while I was in high school. I burned the candle at both ends and only slept a couple hours a night, if that."

We felt sorry for him and, especially, for his daughter. She was only five when he was confined to a wheel chair, and he didn't live long enough to see her graduate from high school.

The Land Sabbaths

But Yahweh also prescribed other kinds of Sabbaths. He designated every seventh year as a *Land Sabbath*, in which the Israelites weren't to do any planting, plowing, or corporate harvesting. Such a practice, when followed, teaches people to plan ahead, store excess produce, and contemplate aspects of their past work, to see if they've been working efficiently.

Yahweh not only planned these Sabbaths to teach His people to depend on Him, but He also wanted them to let the soil rest. Why? Well, even the pagans knew that overworked farmland yields poor results and needs a way to replenish itself. Note this quote from *Ovid*: "Take rest; a field that has rested gives a bountiful crop."

The Israelites weren't told they had to be idle during the Sabbatical year; they could have practiced wood carving, fishing, tent-making – any occupation that would give them a break from working with the soil and let them return to farming with renewed enthusiasm.

When our children were little, we lived on a small farm. Frank loved his garden, but he was always glad when the growing season ended. He spent the winter nights studying the seed catalogs and planning which vegetables he'd plant the following season. He taught or counseled children during the school year and always returned to his garden with renewed zeal when spring rolled around. Imagine how bored the Israelites must have grown after six years of tending barley in the spring, veggies and wheat in the summer, and grapes in the fall.

Every Sabbatical year should have been a year of rejoicing, planning improvements for the next year, and refurbishing plows and garden tools. Instead, the Israelites disobeyed Yahweh's rules for keeping the land fertile and their bodies and spirits refreshed. By the time the Savior walked the streets of Israel, the people's life span had greatly decreased.

When Yahweh announced His plan to let the land rest every seventh year, He warned that if His people *failed* to follow His instructions, He'd allow enemy nations to conquer them, lay the land waste, and allow it to get the rest He planned for it. This is recorded in Leviticus 26:33-35 and also verse 43.

Sure enough, sometime after the people settled in Canaan, the land they'd been promised, they began ignoring these land Sabbaths, and Yahweh kept His word. He allowed two different nations to conquer them. The ten Northern tribes called *Israel,* which departed from His teachings first, were crushed by the Assyrian army. As Yahweh warned, the people were scattered afar and assimilated into other cultures.

The remaining tribes, called *Judah,* obeyed Yahweh's dictates a while longer but were eventually conquered by Babylonians, and many were taken to live in that pagan land. They had to stay in Babylon for seventy years so the overworked land could enjoy its rest. The priests afterward admitted that Judah's seventy years of Babylonian captivity was partly due to this neglect of the land Sabbaths. See 2nd Chronicles 36:20+21.

When the seventy years of captivity ended, many Judean families stayed in Babylon because they had become assimilated into the culture and forsook the worship of Yahweh.

Those who returned to Jerusalem after the seventy years founded a new Israelite nation, but the people started depending on their religious leaders instead of reading *torah* for themselves. To keep the people from falling into idolatry again, the priests and rabbis introduced more rituals and traditions, found in the *Mishnah* and the *Talmud,* which often contradicted the commands Yahweh had dictated to Moses.

By the time the Savior appeared in Israel, the people were steeped in these man-made traditions, and He often corrected them for "not knowing the Scriptures." It's no wonder they suffered from poor health.

In addition to His Land Sabbaths, Yahweh also instituted a special Sabbatical celebration every 50th year. Called a *Jubilee*

Year, it was a time when people were supposed to trust in Him for their food and drink because no crops were to be harvested that year or the year before (every 49th year was a Land Sabbath). The Jubilee year was also a time when slaves were to be freed and rented land was to revert to its original owner.

It's obvious that the majority of Israelites weren't keeping the Land Sabbaths, because the Savior had to remind all his listeners that their Heavenly Father cares for them as lovingly as He cares for each sparrow. If they'd been keeping those Land Sabbaths, they would have experienced — first-hand — the way Yahweh met all their needs; and they wouldn't have needed reminding that Yahweh loves and cares for His own.

Mandated Vacations

Men more interested in conducting business and accumulating wealth will sometimes send the wife and children off for a vacation and try to get more work done while the family is gone. In the same manner, greedy Israelites might have been tempted to send the rest of the family off to receive the spiritual blessing of Yahweh's mandated festivals while they stayed home and made more money.

But Yahweh directly forbade them from doing so; He commanded that all Israelite MALES were to attend His three annual gatherings. Yahweh also planned for them to travel a distance from their homes for these holy convocations, so their minds wouldn't be on their houses and gardens.

Each of these festivals had at least one *High Sabbath,* which Yahweh called a *"holy convocation."* On these Sabbaths, which were different from the weekly Sabbath, they were to congregate in a place where Yahweh was worshipped and where there would be priests available to read *torah* to them.

Although women and children were welcome, these annual appointments were designed for more than just spiritual revival. They were designed for health and rejuvenation, not only spiritually but also physically and mentally.

For instance, during the week-long *Feast of Unleavened Bread,* the people weren't to eat raised bread. Avoiding leaven for seven days is a natural remedy for Candida, which thrives on yeast and is aggravated by sugar and large amounts of wheat.

Seven weeks after the first annual festival came the *Feast of Weeks,* following the wheat harvest. Although this convocation always fell on the first day of the week and provided only a short break from work, the people probably journeyed to Jerusalem, Shiloh, or wherever there was a synagogue, a few days in advance so they wouldn't have to travel on the weekly Sabbath, the day preceding this particular High Sabbath.

Besides Sunday's being the first day of the week, it's also the eighth consecutive day — a number that (in Hebrew thinking) signifies "new beginnings." After observing this feast, the people were to return to their homes physically, mentally, and spiritually refreshed — ready to tackle the fall crops.

The people didn't have to worry about their houses or lands because Yahweh promised that no calamities would befall them or their property while they were attending His holy gatherings. And along the way they'd enjoy friendly discussions with other families about current events and spiritual matters.

In addition to hearing Yahweh's instructions (portions of the *torah*) read each day during the festivals and being reminded of precepts they might have forgotten; the people were required to live simply for a whole week in tents or booths made of tree branches during the week-long *Feast of Tabernacles*. This mandatory vacation assured their getting plenty of fresh air and sunshine following the grape harvest, so those who tended to overwork might get to bed at a decent hour, since they couldn't bring their vineyards with them.

Imagine being able to take three vacations a year with people who believe the same way you do, having your fill of outdoor activities, and not having to worry about leaving your home unattended while you're away!

We'd be a lot healthier if we used our vacation time to get plenty of fresh air and sunshine with adequate sleep every night. To learn more about Yahweh's holy days, which are mentioned at least seven times in the Bible, Leviticus 23 lists them as they appear in Yahweh's annual calendar.

The Israelite wives must have loved these gatherings, too — no one would expect them to prepare elaborate meals while on the road or living in a tent. So they'd have time to enjoy the festivities and socialize with the other women instead of slaving over meals. And speaking of meals –

Chapter 26 — Not Bread!

Wherefore do ye spend money for that which is not bread? And your labour for that which satisfieth not? Hearken diligently unto me and eat ye that which is good, and let your soul delight itself in fatness. — Isaiah 55:2

Years ago, I heard about MSG's ability to stimulate our appetites and make us overeat. So I carefully avoided buying packaged foods with MSG printed on the label. Several years later, I learned that MSG doesn't always go by its chemical name — mono<u>s</u>odium glutamate. The words *natural flavoring* can describe MSG additives, as well as the words *soy isolate* and *hydrolyzed vegetable protein*. And, in fact, Accent® and Natural Meat Tenderizer® are simply MSG products marketed under another name.

After learning that information, we switched to Braggs® Aminos when trying to find a healthful replacement for soy sauce in our recipes. Imagine my dismay when a friend brought to my attention that the FDA ordered Braggs® to remove the words "no MSG" from their label. Although the Braggs® don't *add* MSG to their soybeans, the liquid concentrate contains free glutamates which have caused health issues for those trying to avoid MSG. Also, Dr. Russell Blaylock in his book *Excitotoxins, The Taste That Kills* — and on his videos — claims that all processed, dark-colored taste enhancers should be considered toxic to the neurons in our brains.

MSG can be made several ways. During World War II the Japanese extracted it from sea weed and flavored their soldiers' rations with it, to make the tinned food taste better. In China, MSG is made from soybeans; and in the Philippines, the main ingredient is sugar cane. But in the U.S. — Remember DuPont's® slogan, "Better Living through Chemistry" — the flavoring is made from *bacteria* that have been fermented.

Not only does MSG stimulate our taste buds so that we eat more, but it also damages nerve cells and can cause headaches and nausea. It doesn't take much research to discover that every hydrolyzed protein product (or protein isolate additive) is MSG, regardless of the name given it. Readers can learn more about MSG and its many hidden forms on Dr. Blaylock's website (Blaylock 2008).

After learning that the excitotoxins in MSG have been linked to neurological diseases like Parkinson's, Frank and I decided we could live without MSG's salty flavor and try to eat our food in a more natural state. Observing the direction the food industry in America is headed, we're getting nervous about eating anything sold in a package, especially when we discovered that they're coming up with flavorings that are cheaper and even more inventive than MSG. The newest taste enhancers, touted to be *sweeter than sweet and saltier than salt*, are high-tech chemically-engineered additives manufactured specifically to "fool human taste buds."

Senomyx® — one of the companies working with these taste enhancers — has developed four novel flavors or "taste modulators" for the food, beverage, and ingredient-supply industries. Their spokesperson says these flavor enhancers will "block bitter tastes and thereby improve the taste characteristics of foods, beverages and pharmaceutical products." I'm glad Frank and I are weaning ourselves off processed foods. We're not interested in *tricking* our taste buds into thinking the food tastes better than it actually does.

Pro-lifers may also want to avoid Senomyx®-enhanced foods for ethical reasons as well as health ones. According to a watch-dog organization, the above company uses "human embryonic kidney cells taken from an electively aborted baby to produce those receptors" related to our taste buds (Govt 2011). When the word got out, "the revelation about Senomyx's research techniques motivated Campbell Soup® to sever all relations with Senomyx®." At the time of my research PepsiCo® hadn't, though.

Junk Food's Debut

When I began my research I thought processed foods didn't appear on the scene until after World War II. Wow, was I wrong! Have you ever heard of Seneca?

Seneca lived in 62 AD, while some of Christ's disciples were still alive, and suggested fasting as a way of ridding the body of false cravings. He claimed that after a fast, "you will readily embrace the fresh fruits, vegetables, nuts and seeds, and you can finally break away from the junk."

I wonder if junk foods were sold at McCave, Hunger King, and Sinai Fried Lizzy's. But whoever originally came up

245

with the idea of "doctored" food, we know junk foods existed and were indulged in at the time of the Apostles. And probably in the days of Moses, as well, since the upper class in Egypt consumed rich, sugary desserts and even enjoyed a type of ice cream made from imported ice or snow.

Deadly Delights

Many researchers trace breast, ovarian, and prostate cancers — as well as diabetes — directly back to a diet of highly processed foods. Do you consider yourself an average American? If so, in 2007 you consumed —

- -120 orders of French fries
- - 150 slices of pizza
- - 45 large bags of potato chips

And, after washing the stuff down with 566 cans of soft drinks, Jane and Joe Average topped off their meals with 120 pastries or desserts and — sometime during the day — munched on 190 candy bars (Cutler 2007).

Who reads the tiny-print labels on candy bar wrappers? Not many, probably. And if they did, would they know that hydrogenated and partially hydrogenated oils are really trans-fatty acids that have been shown to cause a buildup of both plaque in our arteries and also toxic amounts of nickel that may cause us kidney, liver, or lung problems?

Would people who see *casein* on a label understand that it's a protein, isolated from cow's milk, to which a majority of adults are allergic? And how about carrageenan, a possible source of added MSG? Carrageenan is a substance added to make liquids feel rich and creamy. Do many people know — or care — that it comes from seaweed that grows only in toxic, polluted water and is believed to cause gastric disturbances?

The Dumbing Down of Americans

But even if we habitually read labels, we need to keep abreast of changes in the food laws. For instance, the FDA will probably give permission for high-fructose corn syrup to be called "natural sweetener" or "corn sweetener" because one of the foods it comes from is corn which, after all, was once a natural food – before it was genetically modified. Also, the makers of Aspartame® keep changing its name when the public begins clamoring about its use in soda pop, chewing gum, and other foods. By the time the public becomes aware of its new name and starts boycotting those products, their makers come out with another moniker for the deadly sweetener.

In addition, the new, previously-mentioned flavor enhancers will be labeled "artificial flavor," and none but those on the lookout will be any wiser.

It's the same with many foods and supplements supposedly safe for vegetarians. One hidden source of animal fat in many packaged foods, including cookies, breads, and pastries, is *mono-and-diglycerides*, an emulsifier and preservative. Unless it's distinctly labeled "vegetable," it's probably derived from an animal fat.

Another byproduct of animals is l-cysteine, often used as a dough conditioner. Although it was originally extracted from human hair, currently duck feathers and animal hairs are used when the human hair supply is short. Vegans steer clear of l-cysteine.

This additive has also been a concern for those who eat a kosher diet, because purchasers could never be sure the hair used to produce the l-cysteine was from a corpse or from a live person (Kashrut.com 2011).

Lying Labelers

Have you ever read on the front of a package of corn chips the words "no trans-fats" only to turn the package over and find *partially hydrogenated oil* listed in the ingredients? We have! We wonder if the producers are stupid, or if they just think *we* are! On the other hand, I believe new regulations allow them to use the "no trans fat" label if the amount of hydrogenated oil is small.

Then there's the newest type of fat making its debut – *interesterified* fat. My understanding is that it consists of separated fats mixed with canola oil, but I haven't seen it on any package labels yet. Maybe manufacturers aren't required to list these fats. But some doctors are worried because *interesterified fats* haven't yet been thoroughly researched for food safety.

Speaking of labeling, even the so-called "vegetarian formula" Vitamin D-3 is falsely labeled, as explained in the osteoporosis chapter. As I stated previously, lanolin from lamb's wool is NOT a vegetable.

For these reasons, Frank and I buy hardly any packaged foods these days. But that doesn't mean we're eating a pure diet!

Foods shipped from California to the East Coast and other distant warehouses are irradiated so they won't spoil in transit and will have a longer shelf life. Formerly, distributers were required to label all produce that was irradiated for commercial use. However, the regulations have been lifted for some; but –

> . . . In other cases, the rule would allow the terms "electronically pasteurized" or "cold pasteurized" to replace the use of "irradiated" on labels. These terms are not used by scientists, but rather are designed to fool consumers about what's been done to their food (Center 2011).

The same source also reported on a 2001 study that "linked colon tumor promotion in lab rats to 2-alkylcyclobu-tanones (2-ACB's), a new chemical compound found only in irradiated foods."

How Do You Like Your Poison?

Have you heard of dioxins? In 1983, United Press International reported that dioxins were the "most deadly substances ever assembled by man . . . 170,000 times as deadly as cyanide." *Chemosphere*, fifteen years later, reported that the primary source of dioxins "for the general population is food, especially meat, fish, and dairy products." And Steve Milloy, author of junkscience.com reported the results of a test on Ben and Jerry's® *World's Best Vanilla Ice Cream* that showed it contained dioxins "200 times greater than the virtually safe dose determined by the Environmental Protection Agency" (Cohen 2011).

Whenever Frank and I have a hankering for ice cream, we just mix ice cubes and frozen bananas in our Vita-Mix® with fresh fruit for sherbet, or with carob powder and sesame seeds for a fudge-flavored delicacy. No unhealthy fats, no animal products, and no hidden sources of dioxins in our ice cream!

Haven't heard of carob powder? It's sometimes called St. John's Bread because it grows on trees, develops into pods like chocolate (often mistranslated in the Bible as "locusts") and is probably the food John the Baptist ate with honey.

Frank and I avoid milk chocolate which contains milk, sugar, and theobromine (a stimulant similar to caffeine). Carob powder requires hardly any sweetening and contains no harmful drugs. In addition, carob helps maintain the alkaline balance in our systems while chocolate creates acidity, thus rendering our bodies more susceptible to disease.

All that Glitters

Over and over, we're told not to judge by appearances because "All that glitters is not gold!" That goes for the produce that looks so good on the grocery shelves too. If tomatoes can be genetically modified by injecting the seeds with DNA from mice, how long will it be before the foods Yahweh originally created have entirely disappeared from the earth?

And if GMO foods are hazardous to our health, as some scientists insist, Yahweh will have to intervene for His people soon, while there are still humans alive on the planet!

In the meantime, we can study the precepts He instituted and try to follow them. It may be that He'll bless our health – in spite of man's tinkering with our food supply – when we show that we trust Him as our primary source of health.

Each of us has to decide whom we'll believe; because –

.

27. Wrap It Up

. . . the Gentiles shall come unto thee from the ends of the earth and shall say, Surely our fathers have inherited lies, vanity, and things wherein there is no profit. — Jeremiah 16:19

The above text describes exactly how I felt when I discovered that the word *torah* doesn't mean the same thing today that it meant when the Bible was written!

And many people feel the same way when they learn that Christ said no part of the *torah* will be changed until heaven and earth pass away (Matthew 5:18). The last time I looked, heaven and earth were still intact. And the medical research — when not tainted or squelched —has affirmed Yahweh's statutes as valid principles for disease-free living.

Short Review

From the research about breast, ovarian, and prostate cancers, we learned that Yahweh's original Genesis diet was designed to ensure optimal health and that He told the patriarchs — including Noah — which flesh foods people could subsist on after the flood so they could remain healthy until the vegetation had time to grow up again. Unfortunately, even the flesh foods once on the "safe-to-eat" list have become so contaminated they are no longer safe to eat, and the return to a plant-based diet is more urgent now than ever before.

We also discovered that Yahweh, being much smarter than we humans, taught principles that have more than one purpose. For instance, the directives about forgiving others and not worrying about the future were designed to give us a sound mind, which has a direct relationship to our physical health.

One of Satan's Wiles

If I were Satan I would try to get Christians hooked on non-nutritious foods so they'd become obese, get sickly and dependent on medications, be no earthly good to anyone, and certainly NOT be the picture of sparkling health and vitality that Yahweh wants His people to be. I would also make them so addicted to their favorite nonfoods that they'd rather believe lies about health and nutrition than change to healthful, life-sustaining habits. The devil hasn't really let me in on his plans, but if that was part of his agenda from the beginning, I'd say he's been very successful!

As Ralph Hodgson said on ESP, "Some things have to be believed to be seen." And that is SO true! Changing our belief system is difficult because we like to hear things that allow us to keep on doing the things we enjoy.

The excuses we've been given for abandoning the guidelines in the *torah* are a great example of our seeing only what we WANT to see. By considering the Old Testament principles to be nonessential for Christendom, church leaders have rendered Yahweh a great disservice and have obscured His promise of health and well-being. How sad that those who claim to believe in Yahweh should suffer all the same diseases and physical ailments that plague nonbelievers!

All Wrapped Up

As stated earlier, Yahweh wants His followers to be physically strong, mentally stable, and spiritually sound. He says, *"If thou wilt diligently hearken to the voice of the Lord thy God, and wilt do that which is right in his sight, and will give ear to his commandments, and keep all his statutes, I will put none of these diseases upon thee, which I have brought upon the Egyptians: for I am the Lord that healeth thee."* (Exodus 15:26)

If we, by faith, claim the above promise in Exodus 15, we should be able to avoid America's lifestyle-related diseases — which also plagued the people of ancient Egypt. We might even reverse many of our present physical ailments.

In closing, I leave you with this blessing from Third John 2, which includes all three areas of wellness: *"Beloved, I wish above all things that thou mayest prosper* [mentally] *and be in health* [physically], *even as thy soul prospereth* [spiritually]."*

Judy Savoy

(Bibliography Follows)

255

Bibliography

7-Steps — www.7-Steps-to-Wellness.com, "Rest: The Pause That Refreshes," retrieved 2/20/11

AAI — *Archives of Allergy Immunology*, March 1998, 115.3

AAKP — American Association of Kidney Patients, http://www.aakp.org/aakp-library/Protein-intake/, retrieved 1/21/11

AARP — http://healthtools.aarp.org/adamcontent/gallbladder-disease?CMP=KNC-360I-GOOGLE-AHBX_PK = gallbladder_disease&utm, retrieved 8/20/10

AARP — http://healthtools.aarp.org/adamcontent/ leprosy? AMP, retrieved 2/21/11 ;

AD — AmazingDiscoveries DVD, a division of Amazing Discoveries®, Walter Veith's Genesis series, 2005; or Dr. McDougall's health segment on AD.tv (2010); or McDougall's website http://www.drmcdougall.com/

ADAA — www.adaa.org/understanding-anxiety/generalized-anxiety-disorder-gad, retrieved 3/28/11

AF — *Amazing Facts* magazine, Roseville, CA 2009, pp. 52-53

AICR — American Institute for Cancer Research 11/09/11

AJCN — *American Journal of Clinical Nutrition*, 1996 Vol. 59 report by Victor Herbert on B-12, pp. 1213S-1222S; 1995; 61; 1994; 59; 1988; 48. 1981, 111; and 1979; 32

AJCN 11/11 — *American Journal of Clinical Nutrition*, November 2011, reported by Robert Cohen

AJE — *American Journal of Epidemiology*, 1995; 142

Akers, Keith, *The Lost Religion of Jesus*, Lantern Books, NY, 2000, p. 164

Allen, Arthur — *Men's health*, 2/16/09, Web MD, article retrieved 6/22/09

Annals of Allergy, 1951; 9   Reported at www.notmilk.com in Dec. 2009

AP — news.yahoo.com/s/ap/20100203/ap, "Report: 40 percent of cancers are preventable," retrieved 2/3/2010

Appleton, Nancy, Ph.D. *Lick the Sugar Habit,* 2004, quoted from Hull's Health Newsletter (See Hull below), retrieved 8/16/10

Archives — *Archives of Internal Medicine*, Vol. 169, No. 6, March 23, 2009

Azur, Beth — Adapted from "Forgiveness helps to keep relationship steadfast," *The APA Monitor,* November 1997, p. 14

Barnard, Neal, *Turn off the Fat Genes*, Three Rivers Press, NY, 2001

Barnard ND, Nicholson A, Howard J, *Preventative Medicine* 1995; 24:646-55 "The medical costs attributable to meat consumption"

Batman — Batmanghelidj, F, M.D. *Your Body's Many Cries for Water*, 1992 and his second book, 2004. Visit http://www.watercure.com/udc.html for more

BBC (2010) — http://www.bbc.co.uk/news, retrieved 9/20/10
BBC (2011) — http://www.bbc.co.uk/news/health-16031149

Believe, 2011 — http://blogs.chron.com/believeitornot/
2011/03/study_prayer_helps_calm_anger.html

Best P — *Best Practice & Research Clinical Gastroenterology*, Vol. 20, No. 6, pp. 997-1015 (2006) available online at www.sciencedirect.com, retrieved June 29, 2010

Blaylock, Dr. — www.russellblaylockmd.com, quotation retrieved from an interview, 2008

BMJ — *British Medical Journal*, 1996; 313

Borland, Sophie, 4/5/11, http://www.dailymail.co.uk/health/ article-1373375/Working 11-hour-day-increase-heart-attack-danger-67-cent.html

Bowdler, Neil, Science reporter, *BBC News*, 10/20/10

Brackett, Neva and Jim, *7 Secrets Cookbook*, Review and Herald Publishing, Hagerstown, MD, 2006, p. 11

British — *British Journal of Cancer*, 83 (1), July 2000

British Medical Journal 1994: 308 and 1996; 313

BTL — *Between the Lines*, Sept. 29, 2000, "Anal Cancer and You," retrieved 8/30/10

Buzzle — http://www.buzzle.com/articles/diseases-caused-by-smoking.html, retrieved 8/23/10

Calif Tissue Int —— a study done at the Calcium Research Institute, Osaka, Japan, 1992

Campbell, T.C, PhD and T.M Campbell II, *The China Study* 2006, Benbella books, Dallas.

Cancer project, *The Survivor's Handbook*, Washington, DC, 2003

CBC News — http://www.cbc.ca/health/stofy/2010/09/09/health-dementia-alzheimer-vitamin-b.html, retrieved 7/16/10

CDC — cdc.gov, Center for Disease Control and Prevention's web site, retrieved 6/22/09, and also quoted in a 2012 news article about the Chesapeake Bay

Center — http://www.centerforfoodsafety.org/campaign/food-irradiation/, retrieved 12/22/11

Circum — http://www.circumcisioninformation.com/index_home_new.html

Chan, J.M., *Seminars in Cancer Biology*, August 1998; 263-73

Clarkson, Priscilla, PhD — http://www.iadms.org/associations/2991/files/info/ dance _nutrition.pdf, 2003-2005

Cohen, Robert, (the Notmilkman), newsletters and articles at http://notmilk.com, 2008-2011

Coresh J., B.C. Astor, T. Greene, G. Eknoyan, and A.S. Levey. "Prevalence of chronic kidney disease and decreased kidney function in the adult US population:" Third National Health and Nutrition Examination Survey. *American Journal of Kidney Disorders* 2003;41:1–12.

Couric, Katie, www.CBSnews/stories/, 2/09/10

CP — *Clinical Pediatrics*, Feb. 1992; Vol. 31 Number 2, pp. 100-104, retrieved 6/22/09

Dark — www.darksideofsleepingpills.com/ by Daniel F. Kripke, M.D., retrieved 7/17/11

Davidson — www.bio.davidson.edu., retrieved 4/27/11

DEAAH — *Department of Environmental and Aquatic Animal Health,* "Research Program and Projects," retrieved online 2/16/09

Despommier, D.D. — www.columbia.edu/cu/21stC/issues, retrieved 5/11/09

Diabetes — American Diabetes Association, www.diabetes.org, retrieved 7/16/10

Diabetologia 2001, 44:63-69. Kimkimaki et al. "Genetic risk . . . Type I diabetes"

Diamond, Harvey, and Marilyn Diamond. *Fit for life,* Warner books, New York, 1985.

Douglass, Herbert E., *Messenger of the Lord* 3rd ed., Pacific Press Publishing Association, Nampa, ID, 1998

Dr. Kim — http://drbenkim.com (1) Article on chronic dehydration, retrieved 2/1/11
Dr. Kim — http://drbenkim.com (2) Articles on processed foods and sleep deprivation/melatonin/cancer, retrieved 2/8/11

Dr. Oz — www.doctoroz.com, retrieved 7/16/10

Easy — received from email@news.easyhealthoptions.com, 5/4/11

EGW — White, Ellen G*., The Upward Look,* Review and Herald Publishing Association, Hagerstown, MD, 1982, p. 102.

Emed — "Normal sleep and sleep deprivation," retrieved 4/4/11 from emedicine's website

Epidemiology 2009 May 20 (3); 355-60)

fitbie — http://fitbie.msn.com/eat-right/tips/6-scary-side-effects-sugar/tip/1, 9/26/11

Fear — http://www.fearofstuff.com/featured/fears-amazing-statistics/, retrieved 3/28/11

Fox — www.foxnews.com/health/2011/01/18/diabetics-diagnosed-breast-cancer-percent-likely-die (results of a study funded by the American Cancer Society)

Franklin — www.fi.edu/learn/brain/exercise.html, retrieved 5/12/11

Gardner, Hanna, M.D., University of Miami Department of Neurology, reporting at the 2011 American Stroke Association's International Stroke Conference in California

Gee W. F. and J. S. Ansell, *Pediatrics* 1976; 58: 824-7, "Neonatal circumcision: A ten-year overview, with comparison of the Gomco clamp and the Plastibell device"

Giles, G. and P. Ireland, *International Journal of Cancer* 1997; Supplement

Goldfarb D.S. and F.L. Coe. "Prevention of recurrent nephrolithiasis." *American Family Physician* 1999;60:2269–76.

Goldschmidt, Vivian, M.A., *The Natural Bone Building Handbook*, ebook, p. 36, retrieved 5/6/2011

Gominak — http://drgominak.com/vitamin-d, 2011

Govt — http://govtslaves.info/2011/05/28/pepsi-uses-aborted-fetal-cells-in-flavor-enhancers/, retrieved 11/19/2011

Greenwood, Carol, Dr., senior scientist at Baycrest in Toronto, in a report made at the Alzheimer'sDisease International Conference, March 26-29, 2011 in Toronto

Guardian — http://www.guardian.co.uk/lifeandstyle/2010/aug/09/breast-cancer-variation, "British say cancer could be prevented by lifestyle," retrieved 8/17/10

Halta website, Ayurvedic medicine. Retrieved 6/22/09

Harvard School of Public Health, published in *The Lancet* Vol. 366; 9499:1784-1793, Nov. 19, 2005

Hautarzt (Germany's Dermatology journal) translated Jan. 17, 2010

Hawker, Dr. David — www.circinfo.com/benefits/bmc.html, retrieved 7/20/10

Health — http://health.yahoo.net/rodale/MH/should-all-males-be-circumcised. 2010

HerbalProvider.com 2009, http://www.herbalprovider.com/liver-disease.html?src=ysm&w=liver-disease&OVRAW=Disease%20Among%20Alcoholic&OVKEY=alcoholic%20liver%20disease%20symptom&OVMTC=advanced&OVADID=55572021511&OVKWID=7302523011&OVCAMPGID=173715011&OVADGRPID=330104399&OVNDID=ND2

Hicks, Gene, *Hope International Newsletter*, Nov.-Dec. 2010

260

Hirshberg — http://www.msnbc.msn.com/id/29777922/ns/health-mens_health/t /should -all-males-be-circumcised/#.T5fjFtn2-Iw, April 2009

Hope-1 — Hope International DVD, May 2010, "The Protein Myth, Part 1" and
Hope-2 — Hope International DVD, May 2011, "The Dangers of Meat Consumption, Part 4"

Horace — *Sermones* i.9.70 (date unknown), quoted on Wikipedia, 2011

Horton, Christine, MD., FACS. www.thdv.com, retrieved 10/09/2007

Hull — Janet Starr's Health Newsletter, December 2003, retrieved 8/16/2010 from http://blpublications.com/html/splendatruth/html

IADM — http://www.iadms.org/displaycommon.cfm?an=1&subarticlenbr=212, 2008

ICGI — http://www.icgi.org/Medicaid_Project/index.htm, as of July 2011

IDN — *Infectious Disease News, Oct. 1997,* "Because of HPV, anal cancer screening indicated for certain high-risk groups"

Iglesias, Antonio A., *The Original Diet*, Richmond, VA, 1998

IGS — http://www.igs.net/~rogersk/tyramine.htm "What is tyramine? Is it harmful?" retrieved 9/26/11

IJE — *International Journal of Epidemiology*, Vol. 26, 657-661 "Modelling the Impact of HIV Disease on Mortality on Gay and Bisexual Men," retrieved Feb. 2009

IJMS — *Israel Journal of Medical Sciences* 1983; 19 (9); 806-809

IN — *Israel News*, www.ynetnews.com, retrieved 11/28/06

Independent — *The Independent* newspaper (Friday 9 June 1995), as well as in the *British Medical Journal* article

JAMA — *Journal of the American Medical Association,* 1995; 272, arterial heart disease

JCO — *Journal of Clinical Oncology,* March 3, 2008

JE — *Jewish Encyclopedia*, 1901-1906 (now in the public domain) "Morbidity"

JER — *Journal of Endocrine Reviews,* article by Clark Grosvenor, 1992, reported by the Notmilkman and retrieved on 12/26/10.

JI — *Journal of Immunology,* April 2001, courtesy of the Notmilkman, 7/13/11

Jiskha — http://www.jiskha.com/spcial_studies/psychology/forgiving.html, retrieved 3/10/11

JNCI — *Journal of the National Cancer Institute* "Diet and Health Study," June 26, 2009

Johnston, Laurance, Ph.D. www.healingtherapies.info/prayer_and_healing, "The science of prayer and healing relevance to physical disability", 2010

Jonsson Cancer Center at UCLA, 2010, www.cancer.ucla.edu

Journal H — *Journal of Health & Longevity,* Vol. 3, (2), Henderson, NV, 2009

Journal of Public Health Nutrition, 2010 Jul 13:1-7

JP — *Jornal de Pedriatria*, a Brazilian journal, February 2007, 83 (1):39-46, retrieved 3/14/11

JRSM — *Journal of the Royal Society of Medicine*, 1985, 78

Kaneshiro, Dennis and Brenda, "None of These Diseases," DVD series, 2010

Kashrut.com — The Premier Kosher Information Source on the Internet, retrieved 4/11/11

Katz, Marc R., M.D. — http://www2.timesdispatch.com/rtd/news/columnists_news/article/BILL10_20100209-210210/323265/

Klotter, Julie, MD., *Townsend Medical Letter,* May 1995

Knight E. L., M. J. Stampfer, S.E. Hankinson, D. Spiegelman, and G.C. Curhan, "The impact of protein intake on renal function decline in women with normal renal function or mild renal insufficiency." *Annals of Internal Medicine* 2003;138:460–7

Koenig — http://www.spiritualityandhealth.duke.edu/about/hkoenig/index.html

Kolonel, Laurence N., MD, PHD, Deputy Director of the Cancer Research Center of Hawaii, quoted in a report by Rebecca Snowden, Nov. 6, 2009

Lambert, Craig, a Pdf document at http://harvardmagazine.com/2005/07/deep-into-sleep.html, retrieved 4/4/11

Lancet, The. Vol. 2, 7160 Nov. 19, 1960 and Vol. 344, November 5, 1994

Larson, Michael F., D.O., Harvard, July 19, 2010, retrieved 8/30/10 from http://emedicine.medscape.com/article/289848-overview

Lee — Dr. Sang Lee, NEWSTART Center, Korea, "Healing by the Word" seminar, 2001

Lindner, Luther, M.D., a pathologist at Texas A & M University, College of Medicine, from his website – courtesy of the Notmilkman, 3/28/11

Lipman — http://www.drfranklipman.com/vitamin-d-faq/, Retrieved 4/22/12

LiveSci — http://www.livescience.com/health/beer-causes-psoriasis-autoimmune-skin-disease-100816.html, retrieved 8/18/10

Livestrong — http://www.livestrong.com/article/238099-high-protein-diet-kidney-problems/, retrieved 1/21/11

Marshall — http://www.marshallprotocol.com/forum39/11446.htm, retrieved 12/4/11

Mayo — http://www.mayoclinic.com/health/rickets/DS00813/DSECTION=sympto, updated Aug. 2011

McMillan, S. I., MD, *None of These Diseases* 1967, Fleming H. Revell Company, NJ.

ME — Ministry of Environment, Victoria, British Columbia, Canada, "Safe and Sensible Pest Control" (brochure). Courtesy of Robert Cohen, 7/8/11

Mead, Nathaniel, M.D., *Natural Health*, July 1994

Medpage 2010 — http://www.medpagetoday.com/Cardiology/MyocardialInfarction/21700 (for the article about bad temper and heart attacks) from original news article at http://abcnews.go.com/Health/MindMoodNews/heart-attack-stroke-prone-arteries-common-nasty-people/story?id=11413859, retrieved 8/18/10

Men's — men's journal website, "A journalist's experience with sleep deprivation," retrieved 4/3/11

Men's Health — By Charles Hirshberg, updated 4/1/2009 8:30:25 AM ET, http://www.msnbc.msn.com/id/29777922/ns/health-mens_health/t/should-all-males-be-circumcised/#.T5crXtn2-Iw

Mental — www.mentalhelp.net/poc/view, retrieved 3/10/11

Mercola, Dr. — http://blpublications.com/html/splendatruth.html Retrieved 8/16/10, See also his article on soda pop, 2011

Miller, G.P., *Virginia Journal of Social Policy and the Law* 2002;9:497-585, "Circumcision: cultural-legal analysis," p. 527

MISH — *Medical Institute of Sexual Health* 1999, "Health Implications Associated with Homosexuality"

Morris, Dr. Brian J., from www.ummah.net/what-is-Islam/misc/, retrieved 7/20/10

MPB — Metro Plus Bangalor, http://www.thehindu.com/mp/2010/01/26/stories/2010012650580400.htm, Online edition of India's National Newspaper, Tuesday, Jan 26, 2010, "Nutrition for those grey cells"

MRB — *Medical Review Board*, 11/14/06, retrieved 6/22/09

Murphy, Frederick A., *Emerging Infectious Diseases*, Vol. 4, No. 3, July-Sept. 1998, University of California, Davis, CA.

NAHL — *Nutrition Action Health Letter*, June 1993

NEJM — *New England Journal of Medicine*, 1992, 326 1173–7

NH — *Natural Health*, "Diabetes Defense," November 2010

NHD — *Natural Health Dossier* online newsletter, Undercover reports for 5/4/11, 5/11/11, and 6/15/11

NIH — National Institute of Health 5/15/10. Reported in an email from www.notmilk.com

Northstar — www.NorthstarNutritionals.com/, retrieved 9/1/11

Notmilkman (See Cohen, above)

NRE — *Neuroepidemiology* 1992;11:30412

Nutrition Action — Healthletter, June, 1993

O'Callaghan, John, ed., *Reuters,* Washington, www.news.yahoo.com 2/8/10

Peck — Dr. Joseph Peck's "Thirty Days to Breakthrough" online journaling seminar series, 2010

Pediatrics-1, "Allergy-Immunology," 1994, 5 (Supplement 5)
*Pediatrics-2, "*Vitamin D overdose," 1963, 31

Peron — James E. "Circumcision: Then and Now". *Many Blessings) (volume III)*: pp.41–42, Spring 2000

Physicians Committee for Responsible Medicine, Washington, D.C. "Health Concerns about Dairy Products," Handout published in 2007

Polish Journal, *Roczniki Akademii Medycznej* 1995: 40 (3)

Psych — www.psychologytoday.com/blog/nourish/201011/amazing-grace

Raji, C.A., et al *Human Brain Mapping*, 2009 August 6, "Brain structure and obesity"

R. G. Stone Urological Research Institute, http://www.rgstoneinternational.com/, retrieved 8/20/10

Righthealth1 — Retrieved on 8/20/10 from video at
    http://www.righthealth.com/topic/Causes_Of_Gall_Bladder_Disease/
Righthealth2 — Retrieved on 8/23/10 from http://www.righthealth.com/topic/Long-term_effects_of_alcohol

Rose, D.P., *Cancer Prevention*, April 9, 2000; 119-23

RR — *Respiratory Research,* June 26, 2009, authored by Fumi Hirayama, Andy H. Lee, and others, and reported by the Notmilkman

Schoen E. J., *Pediatrics* 1993; 92: 860-1, "Circumcision updated?implicated"

Science — http://www.sciencedaily.com/releases/2010/12/101210110703.htm

SciM — *Science* magazine, 1986; 233 (4763)

Secret — Secret report from *Natural Health Dossier,* published online 4/27/2011

SH — *The Survivor's Handbook*, the cancer project, Washington, DC. 2003

Sleep — *Sleep* 31; no. 11, November 2008, 1507-1514; "Associations Between Sleep Duration Patterns and Overweight/Obesity at Age 6."

Smart-heart — www.Smart-heart-living.com/anger-and-heart-disease.html (retrieved 3/8/2011)

Snowden, D. A., R. L. Phillips, and Gary E. Fraser, *Preventative Medicine* 1984:13, 490-500 and quoted in Douglass's book

Spector, Kaye, *The Plain Dealer*, www.cleveland.com/healthy-eating/index   Aug. 4, 2010

Squires, Sally, *Washington Post*, February 27, 2001, page HE10

Thorogood M., J. Mann, P. Appleby, and K. McPherson, *British Medical Journal* 1994; 308:1667-70, "Risk of death from cancer and ischaemic heart disease in meat and non-meat eaters."

Times — http://www2.timesdispatch.com/rtd/news/columnist_news/article /BILL10_20100209-210210/323265/, retrieved 2/28/10, previously appeared in the Richmond, VA, newspaper.

Tracy, Brian, *Maximum Achievement*, Simon & Schuster, NY, 1993, pp. 250-260

Twogood, Daniel, D.C., *No Milk*, Wilhelmina Books, Victorville, CA, 1991

Uic — http://www.uic/edu/classes;osci/osci590/6_2Mummies, "Diseases in Ancient Egypt," Retrieved 5/14//11

US — U.S. Cancer Statistics Working Group. *United States Cancer Statistics: 1999–2007 Incidence and Mortality Web-based Report.* Atlanta (GA): Department of Health and Human Services, Centers for Disease Control and Prevention, and National Cancer Institute; 2010. http://www.cdc.gov/cancer/cervical/statistics/

Van Statan, Michael, M.D., retrieved 8/20/10 from
   http://www.michaelvanstraten.com/factsheets/gall_bladder_problems.pdf

Vegan — *www.vegan.org/FAQs/Index.html*   Retrieved 8/16/2010

Vivo — http://www.vivo.colostate.edu/hbooks/pathphys/endocrine/ otherendo/vitamind.html, Retrieved 4/22/12

WCRF — *World Cancer Research Fund* 1997, American Institute of Cancer Research, Washington, DC, "Food, nutrition and the prevention of cancer. A global perspective."

Webmd — www.webmd.com/balance/features/can-prayer-heal, retrieved 4/7/10

WHO — http://www.who.int/mediacentre/factsheets/fs241/en/, retrieved 4/24/12

Wikipedia – https://en.wikipedia.org/wiki/

Wolbarst, A. L., *JAMA* 1914;62:92-97, "Universal circumcision as a sanitary measure," p. 95

Worry — the worry depository, www.theworrydepository, retrieved 3/28/11

Xiam, Glen L, M.D., 11/23/09 University of California Davis School of Medicine, 8/30/10 from http://emedicine.medscape.com/article/288379-overview

Yahoo1 — http://news.yahoo.com/s/afp/20110116/ts_afp/healthussmoking
Yahoo2 — http://news.yahoo.com/s/yblog_localchi/20110310/ts_yblog_localchi/sleeping-with-your-pet-can-be-unhealthy-study-says. . . .

Your Health website — http://www.pcrm.org/health/reports/highprotein_registry.htm, retrieved 1/21/11

Zodhiates, *The Complete Word Study Old Testament: King James Version*, Warren Baker, editor, AMG Publishers, Chattanooga, TN, 1994.

Zoonoses — *Zoonoses Public Health*, (2011 Jun;58(4):252-61